Advances and Perspectives of Infections Caused by *Staphylococcus aureus*

Edited by Jaime Bustos-Martínez, Juan José Valdez-Alarcón and Aida Hamdan-Partida

Published in London, United Kingdom

Advances and Perspectives of Infections Caused by *Staphylococcus aureus*
http://dx.doi.org/10.5772/intechopen.1003302
Edited by Jaime Bustos-Martínez, Juan José Valdez-Alarcón and Aida Hamdan-Partida

Contributors
Anaid Bustos-Hamdan, Ana Raquel Pereira da Silva, Aída Hamdan-Partida, Cagla Celik, Camila Aparecida Pereira da Silva, Cemile Yilmaz, Dalal Alkuraythi, Damiana Gonçalves de Sousa Freitas, Esma Eryilmaz-Eren, Ismail Ocsoy, Jacqueline Cosmo Andrade-Pinheiro, Jaime Bustos-Martínez, Josefa Sayonara dos Santos, Juan Antonio Guzmán Salgado, Juliete Bezerra Soares, Maria do Socorro Costa, Mehmet Akif Dündar, Nara Juliana Santos Araújo, Nilay Ildiz, Samuel González García, Suhanya Duraiswamy, Sushama Agarwalla, Uner Kayabas, Vanessa Lima Bezerra

First published in London, United Kingdom, 2025 by IntechOpen
IntechOpen is the global imprint of INTECHOPEN LIMITED, registered in England and Wales, registration number: 11086078, 167-169 Great Portland Street, London, W1W 5PF, United Kingdom

For EU product safety concerns: IN TECH d.o.o., Prolaz Marije Krucifikse Kozulić 3, 51000 Rijeka, Croatia, info@intechopen.com or visit our website at intechopen.com.

British Library Cataloguing-in-Publication Data
A catalogue record for this book is available from the British Library

Advances and Perspectives of Infections Caused by *Staphylococcus aureus*
Edited by Jaime Bustos-Martínez, Juan José Valdez-Alarcón and Aida Hamdan-Partida
p. cm.

This title is part of the Infectious Diseases Book Series, Volume 35
Topic: Bacterial Infectious Diseases
Series Editor: Alfonso J. Rodriguez-Morales
Topic Editors: Tomas Jarzembowski and Katarzyna Garbacz

Print ISBN 978-0-85466-887-8
Online ISBN 978-0-85466-886-1
eBook (PDF) ISBN 978-0-85466-888-5
ISSN 2631-6188

If disposing of this product, please recycle the paper responsibly.

IntechOpen Book Series

Infectious Diseases

Volume 35

Aims and Scope of the Series

This series will provide a comprehensive overview of recent research trends in various Infectious Diseases (as per the most recent Baltimore classification). Topics will include general overviews of infections, immunopathology, diagnosis, treatment, epidemiology, etiology, and current clinical recommendations for managing infectious diseases. Ongoing issues, recent advances, and future diagnostic approaches and therapeutic strategies will also be discussed. This book series will focus on various aspects and properties of infectious diseases whose deep understanding is essential for safeguarding the human race from losing resources and economies due to pathogens.

Meet the Series Editor

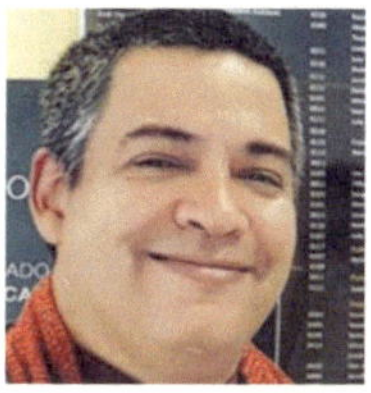

Dr. Rodriguez-Morales is an expert in tropical and emerging diseases, particularly zoonotic and vector-borne diseases (notably arboviral diseases), and more recently COVID-19 and Monkeypox. He is the president of the Publications and Research Committee of the Pan-American Infectious Diseases Association (API), as well as the president of the Colombian Association of Infectious Diseases (ACIN). He is a member of the Committee on Tropical Medicine, Zoonoses, and Travel Medicine of ACIN. Dr. Rodriguez-Morales is a vice-president of the Latin American Society for Travel Medicine (SLAMVI) and a member of the Council of the International Society for Infectious Diseases (ISID). Since 2014, he has been recognized as a senior researcher at the Ministry of Science of Colombia. He is a professor at the Faculty of Medicine of the Fundacion Universitaria Autonoma de las Americas, in Pereira, Risaralda, Colombia, and a professor, Master in Clinical Epidemiology and Biostatistics, at Universidad Científica del Sur, Lima, Peru. He is also a non-resident adjunct faculty member at the Gilbert and Rose-Marie Chagoury School of Medicine, Lebanese American University, Beirut, Lebanon, and an external professor, Master in Research on Tropical Medicine and International Health, at Universitat de Barcelona, Spain. Additionally, an invited professor, Master in Biomedicine, at Universidad Internacional SEK, Quito, Ecuador, and a visiting professor, Master Program of Epidemiology, at Diponegoro University, Indonesia. In 2021 he was awarded the "Raul Isturiz Award" Medal of the API and, the same year, the "Jose Felix Patiño" Asclepius Staff Medal of the Colombian Medical College due to his scientific contributions to the topic of COVID-19 during the pandemic. He is currently the Editor in Chief of the journal Travel Medicine and Infectious Diseases. His Scopus H index is 55 (Google Scholar H index 77) with a total of 725 publications indexed in Scopus.

Meet the Volume Editors

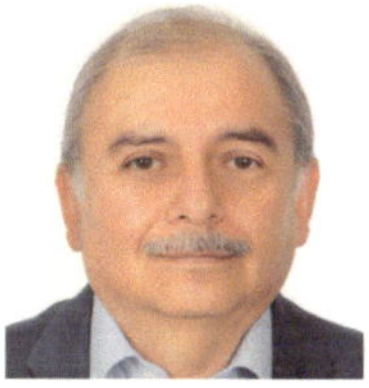

Dr. Jaime Bustos-Martínez is a Research Professor at the Universidad Autónoma Metropolitana-Xochimilco, in Mexico City, Mexico. He has a degree in Biological Pharmaceutical Chemist, an MSc in Biochemical Sciences and a Ph.D. in Biomedical Sciences. For more than 20 years, his field of study has been related to virulence factors, molecular epidemiology and nanoparticles against Staphylococcus aureus. His studies have been published in several articles in indexed journals and presented in international forums. He has written several chapters of textbooks, as well as divulgation. He is a reviewer for multiple recognized journals. He is part of the National System of Researchers in Mexico.

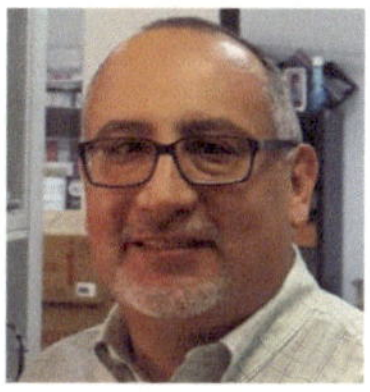

Dr. Juan José Valdez Alarcón is a Research Professor at the Faculty of Veterinary Medicine and Animal Production in the Multidisciplinary Centre of Studies in Biotechnology at the Universidad Michoacana de San Nicolás de Hidalgo in Michoacán, Mexico. As a microbiologist with a Ph.D. in Biotechnology, focused on Molecular Epidemiology and Biotechnology, he approaches to study and control bacterial diseases in animals. He has published over 60 research and divulgation papers in national and international scientific journals and 9 book chapters. He has also collaborated as a member of the advisory committee of national and international scientific meetings, reviewer of microbiology topics for well-recognized scientific journals, and currently as Coordinator of the Animal Microbiology Network of the Microbial and Invertebrates Genetic Resources Subcommittee of the Agricultural and Rural Development Secretary in México.

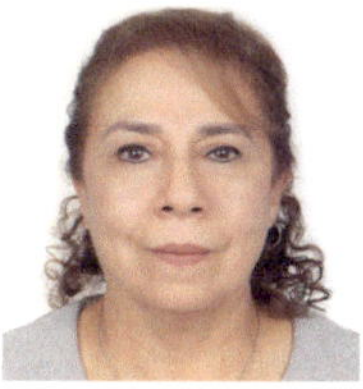

Dr. Aída Hamdan-Partida is a professor-researcher at the Department of Health Care at the Universidad Autónoma Metropolitana Xochimilcon in Mexico City, Mexico. She holds a bachelor's degree in Biological Pharmaceutical Chemistry, a master's degree in Biotechnology and a Ph.D. in Biological and Health Sciences. She has worked in the pharmaceutical industry, and her field of research is microbiology, especially regarding S. aureus. She is currently investigating new methods to combat it using nanoparticles. She has published several articles in indexed journals and book chapters. She has directed several bachelor and doctoral theses. She belongs to the National System of Researchers of Mexico.

Contents

Preface

Staphylococcus aureus is one of the few species of the genus *Staphylococcus* that is coagulase-positive and an important pathogen of humans and mammals.

S. aureus can colonize around 30% of the population, mainly in the nose, pharynx, skin and other parts of the human body. Under certain conditions, it can pass from a commensal, non-pathogenic state to an infectious agent state, causing infections ranging from mild to life-threatening.

Two main types of strains are recognized, methicillin-sensitive *S. aureus* (MSSA) and methicillin-resistant *S. aureus* (MRSA). The latter are the strains that cause the most health problems. Their pathogenic capacity lies in the large number of virulence factors they present and their ability to acquire antibiotic resistance, so they are considered a multidrug-resistant (MDR) bacteria. Because of this, the World Health Organization places methicillin-resistant *Staphylococcus aureus* as a high-priority microorganism in its most recent list of priority bacterial pathogens for the year 2024.

Within the MRSA strains, there are genetically typed as hospital-acquired MRSA strains (HA-MRSA), community-acquired MRSA (CA-MRSA) and livestock-acquired MRSA (LA-MRSA). The first was found in hospitals in the 1960s; the second appeared in the 1990s in people in the community who had not been hospitalized, and the third type appeared on farms in the middle of the first decade of the 21st century.

Currently, HA-MRSA strains have spread from hospitals to the community, and CA-MRSA strains from the community have entered hospitals. In addition, LA-MRSA strains have begun to spread from animals to humans and vice versa.

This variety of strains with different characteristics and their dissemination processes, together with all the genetic recombination mechanisms, have led to the implementation of extensive epidemiological surveillance of this bacterium, as well as the in-depth study of all the virulence mechanisms it presents, including adhesion proteins, toxins, biofilm formation and resistance to antibiotics, among many other factors. The search for new compounds to combat this microorganism has also increased.

For all these reasons, we decided to make a contribution to the study of *Staphylococcus aureus* in this publication, where through several chapters, relevant aspects of its virulence and pathogenicity factors are discussed, and an important factor in infections by this microorganism, which is the formation of biofilms, is also reviewed. Another critical and determining aspect in diagnosing and treating this bacteria is its rapid and efficient detection and genotyping, which is discussed in one of the chapters.

Furthermore, knowing the type of strains found in the community, it is essential to provide adequate treatment and implement prevention and disinfection programs; an example of this is shown in one of the chapters.

Finally, the perspectives regarding infections caused by *Staphylococcus aureus* are presented.

We hope you enjoy this book and find relevant information in the study of *Staphylococcus aureus*.

Dr. Jaime Bustos-Martínez and Dr. Aída Hamdan-Partida
Department of Health Care,
Autonomous Metropolitan University-Xochimilco,
Mexico City, Mexico

Dr. Juan José Valdez-Alarcón
Faculty of Veterinary Medicine and Zootechnics,
Multidisciplinary Center for Studies in Biotechnology,
Universidad Michoacana de San Nicolás de Hidalgo,
Michoacán, Mexico

Chapter 1

Virulence Factors and Pathogenicity of *Staphylococcus aureus*

Dalal Alkuraythi

Abstract

This chapter will explore the virulence factors and pathogenicity mechanisms of *Staphylococcus aureus*, a major human pathogen responsible for a wide range of infections. It will provide a detailed analysis of the key virulence factors, including surface proteins like adhesins and Protein A, various exotoxins such as alpha-toxin and Panton-Valentine leukocidin (PVL), and important enzymes like coagulase and hyaluronidase. The chapter will also examine how these factors contribute to immune evasion, tissue damage, and the formation of biofilms, leading to chronic and healthcare-associated infections. By understanding these mechanisms, we can better combat *S. aureus* infections and reduce their significant global health impact.

Keywords: Panton-Valentine leukocidin (PVL), toxic shock syndrome toxin (TSST-1), enterotoxins, coagulase, hyaluronidase, virulence factors, pathogenicity, adhesins, protein A, immune evasion, biofilm formation, Agr systems

1. Introduction

Staphylococcus aureus is an important bacterial pathogen that affects humans and causes a variety of clinical manifestations [1]. It is the world's most significant opportunistic human pathogen, known for its ability to bypass the immune system and cause various infections [2]. Commonly found in the human microbiota, *S. aureus* colonizes various sites within the human body, particularly in the nasal area, but also including the skin, throat, and gastrointestinal tract [3].

While it typically does not cause infections, *S. aureus* can lead to severe infections if it penetrates the skin and enters the bloodstream or internal tissues [4]. *S. aureus* infections range from mild skin and tissue infections to life-threatening conditions such as endocarditis, chronic osteomyelitis, pneumonia, and bacteremia, all of which are associated with serious morbidity and high mortality [5]. Many of these infections are iatrogenic, often linked to the colonization of indwelling medical devices [6]. The body's inflammatory response, triggered by macrophages and cytokines, summons neutrophils to the site of infection following bacterial invasion [7]. The primary method of managing *S. aureus* infections is through the defense mechanisms of the human body, primarily phagocytosis by specialized phagocytes like macrophages and neutrophils [8]. However, *S. aureus* has developed several strategies to evade the immune response [8]. To survive and adapt to various environmental niches, *S. aureus* has evolved a complex regulatory network for controlling virulence factor production in a temporal and host-specific manner [9]. These virulent factors enable the organism to evade host defenses, bind to cells and tissue matrices, disseminate within hosts, and degrade tissues and cells for survival and nourishment [10]. The molecular pathogenesis of staphylococcal infections involves a myriad of mechanisms and factors that underscore the bacterium's adaptability and virulence [11].

2. *Staphylococcus aureus* virulent factors and pathogenicity

2.1 The ability to adhere to host cells and resist physical removal

2.1.1 Collagen adhesin protein (Cna) is encoded by the cna gene

Collagen adhesin protein is a crucial virulence factor in *S. aureus* [12]. A critical step in initiating and persisting in multiple bacterial infections is the bacterial adhesion to collagen, the most abundant protein in humans [12]. This adhesion is vital for *S. aureus* to establish infections, particularly in collagen-rich tissues such as joints, bones, and heart valves, leading to conditions like osteomyelitis, septic arthritis, and endocarditis [13]. The *cna* gene, which encodes collagen adhesin, belongs to the microbial surface components recognizing adhesive matrix molecules (MSCRAMM) family and is not present in every strain of *S. aureus* [14]. The encoded protein comprises an N-terminal signaling peptide, a non-repetitive (A region), multiple repeated units (B region), a cell wall anchor region, a transmembrane section, and a small, positively charged cytoplasmic tail [12]. The A region of Cna is entirely responsible for its collagen-binding activity, making it a key factor in the pathogen's ability to adhere to and invade host tissues [13]. This binding facilitates the colonization and subsequent infection of the host, contributing to the bacterium's ability to evade the immune system and persist within the host [8]. The presence of Cna enhances the pathogenicity of *S. aureus* by enabling it to anchor to host tissues, resist phagocytosis, and form biofilms [15]. Biofilms provide a protective environment for the bacteria, increasing their resistance to antibiotics and the host immune response [15]. By integrating these mechanisms, *S. aureus* can cause chronic and recurrent infections, highlighting the importance of Cna as a virulence factor [12]. Understanding the role of collagen adhesin protein in *S. aureus* pathogenicity is essential for developing targeted therapies to prevent and treat infections caused by this formidable pathogen.

2.1.2 Clumping factors encoded by the clfA and clfB genes

These genes are part of the microbial surface components recognizing the adhesive matrix molecules (MSCRAMM) family [16]. Clumping factor proteins A (ClfA) and B (ClfB) facilitate the pathogen's adhesion to host tissues by binding to the blood plasma protein fibrinogen (Fg), with ClfA targeting the γ-chain and ClfB the α-chain [16]. This differential binding enhances *S. aureus*' ability to form clumps, resist immune clearance, and establish infections [17]. ClfA, in particular, plays a crucial role in *S. aureus*-induced platelet aggregation, contributing to the pathogen's ability to cause severe bloodstream infections [2]. The *clf*A and *clf*B genes are distinct, non-allelic, and not closely linked, unlike other MSCRAMM-encoding genes such as *fnb*A and *fnb*B [18]. These clumping factors promote bacterial aggregation, biofilm formation, and resistance to both immune defenses and antibiotics, significantly enhancing *S. aureus* pathogenicity [19].

2.1.3 Fibronectin-binding proteins (FnBPs) encoded by the fnbA and fnbB genes

These proteins, FnBPA and FnBPB, facilitate the formation of biofilms on indwelling medical devices such as central venous catheters and prosthetic joints [20]. Biofilm-associated infections are particularly challenging to treat with antibiotics due to the dormant state of many cells within the biofilm matrix [21]. Most strains of *S. aureus* produce two similar fibronectin-binding proteins, FnBPA and FnBPB, encoded by closely linked genes [18]. The aforementioned proteins are a member of the MSCRAMM family, which are proteins on the cell surface that binds to both fibrinogen and fibronectin [22]. In methicillin-resistant *S. aureus* (MRSA) strains, FnBPs play a key role in biofilm formation, enhancing the bacterium's ability to persist in the host and resist antibiotic treatment [23]. FnBPs bind to fibronectin in the extracellular matrix (ECM), which in turn interacts with the $\alpha5\beta1$ integrin on host cells through the Arg-Gly-Asp (RGD) motif in fibronectin [24]. This interaction forms a bridge between *S. aureus* and host cell integrins, facilitating bacterial adherence and colonization [24]. By promoting biofilm formation and mediating adhesion to host tissues, FnBPs significantly enhance the pathogenicity of *S. aureus*, making infections difficult to eradicate [24].

2.1.4 Elastin-binding protein of Staphylococcus aureus *(EbpS) encoded by ebp gene*

Elastin, a crucial component of the elastic fiber extracellular matrix (ECM) along with microfibrillar elements, is abundant in tissues requiring elasticity, such as the heart, skin, and major blood vessels [25]. It consists of tropoelastin monomers, which are cross-linked by modified lysine side chains and deposited in tissues [25]. *S. aureus* expresses elastin-binding protein (EbpS) as an integral membrane protein on the cell surface, rather than as a cell-wall-associated protein [15]. EbpS specifically attaches to the N-terminal region of elastin, promoting the attachment of soluble elastin peptides and tropoelastin to *S. aureus* cells [26]. However, EbpS does not facilitate bacterial adherence to immobilized elastin and, therefore, is not considered a microbial surface component recognizing adhesive matrix molecule (MSCRAMM) [26]. This selective binding capability aids *S. aureus* in colonizing and infecting elastic tissue-rich environments, contributing to its pathogenicity in host tissues that require elasticity [17].

2.1.5 Serine-aspartate repeat-containing protein (Sdr) encoded by sdrC, sdrD, and sdrE genes

Sdr proteins (from SD Repeat) are characterized by an R region with multiple serine-aspartate repeats [27]. The *sdr* locus in *S. aureus* encodes three proteins: SdrC, SdrD, and SdrE [28]. While SdrC is consistently present, SdrD and SdrE are variably found, with SdrE linked to more invasive strains [28]. These proteins, part of the MSCRAMM family, primarily bind to bone sialoprotein and fibrinogen, enhancing *S. aureus*' adhesion to host tissues [13]. This adhesion facilitates biofilm formation, protects the bacteria from immune responses and antibiotics, and is crucial in infections involving bones and blood vessels [19]. By promoting biofilm formation and aiding in tissue colonization, Sdr proteins significantly contribute to *S. aureus* pathogenicity, making the bacterium more adept at establishing and maintaining infections [19].

2.1.6 The extracellular adherence protein (Eap), AKA major histocompatibility class II analogous protein (Map), encoded by map gene

The extracellular adherence protein (Eap), also known as major histocompatibility class II analogous protein (Map), is encoded by the *map* gene. Unlike MSCRAMM proteins that are cell surface-bound, Eap is a secreted protein classified as a Secreted Expanded Repertoire Adhesive Molecule (SERAM) [13]. Eap plays a crucial role in *S. aureus* pathogenesis by aiding bacterial adherence and evading host defenses [29]. Eap binds strongly to extracellular matrix proteins such as fibrinogen, fibronectin, bone sialoprotein, vitronectin, and thrombospondin, enhancing bacterial adhesion and promoting chronic infections [13]. It also has a high tendency to form oligomers, leading to *S. aureus* aggregation [30]. Additionally, Eap can interact with intercellular adhesion molecule-1 (ICAM-1), modulating the inflammatory response and contributing to the pathogen's ability to persist in the host [30]. Overall, Eap significantly contributes to the virulence of *S. aureus* by facilitating bacterial adhesion, promoting aggregation, and interfering with host immune responses [30].

2.1.7 Intercellular adhesion proteins encoded by the icaA, icaB, icaC, icaD, and icaR genes

The most important virulence factor of *S. aureus* bacteria is their capability to attach and form biofilms [13]. The *ica*ADBC gene locus is essential for synthesizing polysaccharide intracellular adhesion (PIA), also known as poly-N-acetyl-β-(1–6)-glucosamine (PIA/PNAG), which contributes to biofilm formation and adherence [31]. The *ica*R gene negatively regulates this locus. IcaA and IcaD function as glucosyltransferases that produce short PIA/PNAG oligomers [31]. IcaC helps bind these oligomers into longer polymer chains and is involved in their transport to the cell surface [31]. On the surface, IcaB facilitates the partial deacetylation of PIA/PNAG, which is crucial for maintaining biofilm integrity and surface adhesion [31]. These proteins collectively enhance *S. aureus'* ability to adhere to surfaces and form biofilms, significantly contributing to its pathogenicity by protecting the bacteria from host immune responses and antibiotic treatment [13].

2.1.8 Staphylokinase (plasminogen activator) is encoded by the sak gene

Staphylokinase interacts with host plasminogen to form active plasmin, a proteolytic enzyme that degrades the extracellular matrix, facilitating bacterial penetration and tissue invasion [30]. This enhances the spread and proliferation of *S. aureus* [30]. Staphylokinase also binds to alpha-defensins, human neutrophil-derived bactericidal peptides, neutralizing their antimicrobial properties [32]. This interaction helps *S. aureus* resist innate immune defenses, making staphylokinase crucial for bacterial survival and virulence [32].

DOI: http://dx.doi.org/10.5772/intechopen.1006633

2.2 The ability to resist innate immune defenses (antiphagocytosis)

2.2.1 Capsule encoded by cap5 and cap8 genes

Capsular polysaccharides (CP) in *S. aureus* are key virulence factors [33]. While older literature suggested up to 11 serotypes, only serotypes 1, 2, 5, and 8 have been chemically characterized [34]. Notably, 75–80% of human isolates belong to CP types 5 (CP5) or 8 (CP8) [35]. The capsule helps *S. aureus* evade the immune system by masking surface proteins and opsonins, preventing recognition by phagocytic cells [36]. Additionally, the secretion of extracellular fibrinogen-binding protein (Efb) further inhibits phagocytic uptake, enhancing the bacterium's ability to persist and cause infections [36].

2.2.2 Cardiolipin synthase is encoded by cls1 and cls2 genes

Cardiolipin synthase converts phosphatidylglycerol (PG) to cardiolipin (CL), a crucial phospholipid in staphylococcal membrane [37]. The alteration of the bacterial membrane composition, particularly the increase in CL, helps *S. aureus* evade last-line antibiotics like daptomycin by impairing their membrane penetration [37]. Additionally, these membrane changes reduce neutrophil chemotaxis, aiding the bacteria in evading phagocytosis and enhancing its pathogenicity [37].

2.3 The ability to evade adaptive immune defenses (immune evasion)

2.3.1 Adenosine synthase (AdsA) is encoded by the adsA gene

S. aureus is a human pathogen that produces extracellular adenosine to evade the host immune system, primarily through the adenosine synthase (AdsA) 5′-nucleotidase function [38]. In mammals, adenosine triphosphate (ATP) is converted to adenosine via a two-step process: ecto-nucleoside triphosphate diphosphohydrolases (Ecto-NTDPases) hydrolyze ATP and ADP into AMP, and 5′ nucleotidases hydrolyze AMP into adenosine, with the activity dependent on Apyrase conserved regions (ACRs) [39]. When *S. aureus* infects host tissues, it releases two enzymes, nuclease and AdsA. Nuclease degrades neutrophil extracellular traps (NETs) DNA into deoxyadenylate (dAMP), which is subsequently converted by AdsA into 2′-deoxyadenosine (dAdo) [8]. dAdo activates the Caspase-3 pathway, inducing macrophage apoptosis [8]. Consequently, *S. aureus* restricts macrophage infiltration into abscess communities, preventing phagocytosis and leading to recurrent and persistent infections [38].

2.3.2 Chemotaxis inhibitory protein of Staphylococcus (CHIPS) encoded by chp gene

Chemotaxis inhibitory protein (CHIPS) plays a crucial role in evading the host's first line of defense [40]. It inhibits the response of human neutrophils and monocytes to complement anaphylatoxin C5a and formylated peptides, such as N-formylmethionyl-leucyl-phenylalanine (fMLP) [41]. CHIPS achieves this by binding directly to the C5a receptor (C5aR) and the formylated peptide receptor (FPR), thereby blocking the calcium responses induced by C5a and fMLP. This action prevents bacterial phagocytosis by leukocytes [41].

2.3.3 Staphylococcal complement inhibitor (SCIN) encoded by scn gene

S. aureus mitigates the host immune response by excreting staphylococcal complement inhibitor (SCIN) residues [42]. SCIN reduces the activity of central complement convertases, thereby decreasing phagocytosis after opsonization and eliminating downstream effector activities [41]. SCIN molecules (SCIN, SCIN-B, and SCIN-C) specifically block C3 convertases (C4b2a and C3bBb) to prevent the generation of C3b/iC3b, phagocytosis, and C5a formation [43]. SCIN does not directly bind to C3b but instead binds to the activated C3 convertase, leading to the stabilization and inactivation of this complex [43].

2.3.4 Staphylococcal protein A (SpA) is encoded by the spa gene

Evasion of the host immune system is integral to *S. aureus'* pathogenicity and is facilitated by the cell wall-associated protein A (SpA) [44]. SpA binds to the Fc fragments of immunoglobulin G (IgG), preventing phagocytosis and classical pathway complement fixation [45]. Both the innate and adaptive immune systems are impaired by SpA, which belongs to the MSCRAMM family [8]. SpA interacts with both the Fc and Fab parts of immunoglobulins to counteract antibody-mediated opsonophagocytic processes and induce the expansion and apoptotic destruction of B-cell populations [46]. Additionally, SpA mediates the attachment of *S. aureus* to von Willebrand factor (VWF), a protein present at sites of endothelial damage, potentially playing a role in the initiation of intravascular infections [47].

2.3.5 Staphylococcal binder of immunoglobulin (Sbi) encoded by the sbi gene

S. aureus' second immunoglobulin-binding protein (Sbi) has two N-terminal domains that bind the IgG Fc region similarly to protein A, and two domains that bind to the C3 complement, facilitating its futile consumption in the fluid phase [44]. Sbi, a 436-amino acid protein associated with the bacterial envelope, contains one functional immunoglobulin-binding domain and a second immunoglobulin-binding motif, both similar to the five immunoglobulin-binding repeats (E, A, B, C, and D) of SpA [48]. Sbi forms a tripartite complex with complement factor C3d and factor H, leading to the consumption of C3 and inhibiting the pathogen's opsonophagocytic clearance [49].

2.4 The ability to compete for iron and other nutrients (iron uptake)

2.4.1 Iron-regulated surface determinant (Isd) series of proteins encoded by isdA, isdB, isdC, isdD, isdE, isdF, isdG, isdH, isdI, and srtB genes

The iron-regulated surface determinant (*isd*) cluster of genes was first identified in 2002, with Hazmanian et al. proposing in 2003 that the Isd protein series forms a heme transport pathway across the cell wall and membrane [50]. In *S. aureus*, the Isd system comprises nine iron-regulated proteins: IsdA, IsdB, IsdC, and IsdH/HarA, which are cell wall-anchored surface proteins; IsdDEF, a membrane-localized transporter; and IsdG and IsdI, heme-degrading cytoplasmic enzymes [50]. This sequence of Isd proteins interacts with heme proteins, extracts the heme molecule, and transfers it through the cell wall to the membrane, where it is translocated to the cytoplasm [51].

2.5 The ability to disseminate and spread the infection (exoenzymes, secretion system)

2.5.1 Aureolysin is encoded by aur gene

S. aureus secretes a metalloproteinase known as aureolysin, encoded by the *aur* gene, which exists in two allelic forms: type I and type II [52]. In vitro, aureolysin degrades plasma proteinase inhibitors, α1-antichymotrypsin and α1-proteinase, and activates prothrombin in human plasma. It also influences T and B lymphocyte stimulation by polyclonal activators and inhibits lymphocyte immunoglobulin production [30]. Additionally, aureolysin activates the glutamyl endopeptidase precursor (V8 protease), also synthesized by *S. aureus* By specifically inactivating ClfB via cleavage of its N-terminal domain, aureolysin modulates bacterial cell surface proteins, facilitating bacterial cell detachment from colonized sites and promoting the infectious spread of the organism [53].

2.5.2 Hyaluronate lyase is encoded by the hysA gene

The enzyme hyaluronate lyase (HL), a long-neglected potential virulence determinant of *S. aureus*, is an extracellular enzyme that degrades the mucopolysaccharide hyaluronic acid (HA), the major intercellular component in human and animal connective tissue [54]. HL removes the 1,4-glycosidic bond between D-glucuronic acid residues and N-acetyl-β-D-glucosamine in hyaluronan, leading to the secretion of unsaturated polysaccharides [54]. The key end product of this process is 2-acetamido-2-deoxy-3-O-(β-D-gluco-4-enepyranosyluronic acid)-D-glucose [54].

2.5.3 Lipase is encoded by the geh gene

The lipase enzyme (glycerol ester hydrolase, EC 3.1.1.3) interacts with host granulocytes, enhancing bacterial survival by inhibiting bactericidal lipids [55]. It releases significant amounts of fatty acids, particularly octadecenoic acid, in human plasma [56]. Lipases support the survival of *S. aureus* in the fatty secretions of mammalian skin, indirectly contributing to its pathogenicity. The expression of lipase-encoding genes is also directly induced during infection, underscoring their role in bacterial virulence [55].

2.5.4 Glutamyl endopeptidase precursor (V8 protease) is encoded by the sspA gene

The enzyme glutamyl endopeptidase, also known as V8 protease preferably cleaves peptide bonds on the carboxyl-terminal side of aspartate and glutamate [57]. This enzyme plays a crucial role in the invasion and infection of human tissues [57]. Together with other extracellular proteases, it is needed for the proteolytic development of SspB thiol protease and the inactivation of SspC, an inhibitor of SspB. V8 protease is the most essential degrading protease of fibronectin-binding protein (FnBP) and surface protein A, both of which are involved in the attachment of *S. aureus* to host cells [58]. Additionally, it may defend bacteria against host protection by cleaving the immunoglobulins IgG, IgA, and IgM, and may also contribute to the stabilization of lipase secretion [59].

2.5.5 Cysteine protease (staphopain) A encoded by scpA and B encoded by sccpB genes, cysteine proteinase inhibitor (staphostatins) encoded by scpC and sspC genes

Cysteine protease is a critical virulence factor in *S. aureus*, playing a significant role in evading the host's innate immune response [30]. It cleaves elastin in connective tissues, pulmonary surfactant protein A in the lungs, and the chemokine receptor CXCR2 in leukocytes [60]. By degrading surfactant protein A, cysteine protease inhibits neutrophil bacterial phagocytosis, and by targeting CXCR2, it prevents neutrophil activation and chemotaxis [60]. This dual action significantly hampers the host's ability to mount an effective immune response against the bacterium [61]. Additionally, staphostatins, which suppress staphopain cysteine protease by blocking its active site, are essential for protecting cytoplasmic proteins from premature degradation [60]. These proteases are associated with bacterial growth, viability, and morphology, further contributing to the pathogen's ability to cause persistent and recurrent infections [30].

2.5.6 Staphylocoagulase is encoded by the coa gene and the von Willebrand factor binding protein is encoded by the vWbp gene

Coagulation is a key innate defense mechanism that captures and immobilizes bacterial pathogens in a clot [7]. *S. aureus* exploits this process through two primary virulence factors: coagulase and von Willebrand factor binding protein (vWbp) [7]. Coagulase, a polypeptide produced by *S. aureus*, binds to and activates prothrombin, which converts fibrinogen into fibrin [62]. This activation promotes blood clotting and facilitates the formation of abscesses, aiding in the pathogen's survival and contributing to severe infections such as lethal bacteremia [62]. Similarly, vWbp functions as an additional coagulase, enabling the bacteria to form thromboembolic lesions [63]. This not only assists in bacterial dissemination but also helps *S. aureus* evade opsonophagocytic clearance by host immune cells, thereby enhancing its ability to persist in the host and cause chronic infections [63].

2.5.7 ESAT-6 secretion system (ESS) (AKA type VII secretion system (T7SS)) encoded by esaA, esaB, esaD, esaE, esaG1-9, essA, essB, essC, esxA, esxB, esxC, and esxD genes

The ESAT-6 secretion system (ESS) in *S. aureus* is essential for its virulence and persistence in infections, such as murine abscesses, pneumonia, and chronic infections in cystic fibrosis patients [64]. The ESS consists of six components: EsxA (a secreted WXG100 protein), EsaB (a regulatory protein), EssC (a membrane protein crucial for secretion), and other transmembrane proteins (EssA and EssB) [65]. EsxA and EsxB contribute significantly to virulence by promoting bacterial dissemination and colonization, and their absence leads to significantly reduced virulence [65]. The T7SS also secretes a nuclease toxin, EsaD, whose activity is regulated by binding to the antitoxin EsaG [66]. Other components such as EsaB, which has a ubiquitin-like fold, regulate the ESS machinery, and membrane proteins EssA, EssB, and EssC facilitate the secretion process [66]. This system is vital for *S. aureus's* ability to evade the host immune system and establish persistent infections [66].

DOI: http://dx.doi.org/10.5772/intechopen.1006633

2.6 Toxins

2.6.1 Hemolysins: α-hemolysin encoded by the hly/hla gene, β-hemolysin encoded by the hlb gene, δ-hemolysin encoded by the hld gene, γ-hemolysin encoded by hlgA, hlgB, and hlgC genes

α-Hemolysin is a hydrophilic protein of approximately 33 kDa that assembles into a heptameric pre-pore complex upon integration with the target cell membrane [67]. This complex forms a β-barrel channel consisting of 14 anti-parallel β-strands, with each protomer contributing two strands [67]. By binding to the ADAM10 receptor on alveolar epithelial cells, α-hemolysin enhances ADAM10 metalloprotease activity, leading to E-cadherin cleavage and subsequent pore formation [68]. This disruption impairs neutrophil function and triggers cytokine release [68]. In contrast, β-Hemolysin, a neutral sphingomyelinase, hydrolyzes sphingomyelin in the plasma membrane to generate phosphocholine and ceramide, essential for its hemolytic activity [69]. δ-Hemolysin destabilizes cell membranes through pore formation, membrane curvature alteration, or solubilization at high concentrations [70]. The phenol-soluble modulins (PSMs) family, including δ-hemolysin and PSMα peptides, contribute to *S. aureus* virulence by disrupting host cell membranes [71]. γ-Hemolysin, consisting of HlgA, HlgB, and HlgC, mimics leukocidins by forming pores in host cell membranes, aiding in bacterial survival and immune evasion [71].

2.6.2 Panton-Valentine leucocidin (PVL) is encoded by lukS-PV and lukF-PV genes

The toxin, known as Panton-Valentine leukocidin (PVL), is composed of two components: LukS-PV and LukF-PV [67]. These components are synthesized separately and then combined to form a heptameric pore on neutrophil membranes, leading to neutrophil lysis [67]. PVL is part of the synergohymenotropical toxin family, which includes γ-hemolysin and other leukocidins such as LukE-LukD [72]. PVL induces cell activation through Ca^{2+} influx and pore formation, which occurs in two successive and independently inhibitable steps [72].

2.6.3 Exfoliative toxin encoded by eta and etb genes

Exfoliative toxins (ETs) are high-substrate-specific serine proteases that selectively target and hydrolyze desmosomal proteins in the skin [73]. Specifically, ETD and ETA are responsible for the skin manifestations seen in staphylococcal scalded skin syndrome and bullous impetigo [73]. These toxins act as serine proteases, with Dsg-1 (desmoglein-1) being their primary target [53]. Dsg-1 is crucial for maintaining cell-to-cell adhesion among keratinocytes [53]. When ETs cleave Dsg-1, it disrupts this adhesion, leading to the separation of keratinocytes and the resultant epidermal tissue layer separation characteristic of these skin conditions [74]. Additionally, ETs may also act as potential superantigens [74].

2.6.4 Toxic shock syndrome toxin-1 (TSST)-1 is encoded by the tsst-1 gene

The *tsst*-1 gene encodes a 21.9 kDa extracellular toxin that induces cytokine secretion from epithelial cells, antigen-presenting cells (APCs), and T lymphocytes, leading to toxic shock syndrome (TSS) [75]. Acting as a superantigen, it triggers

T-cells by binding the variable portion of the β-chain of the T-cell receptor to major histocompatibility complex class I molecules on target T-cells outside the peptide-binding groove [76]. This results in the massive, non-specific activation of T-cells, significantly contributing to the pathogenicity of *S. aureus* [76].

2.6.5 Staphylococcal enterotoxin (SE) is encoded by sea, seb, sec1, sec3, sed, see, seh, selk, and selq genes

Staphylococcal enterotoxins (SEs) are superantigens primarily responsible for the symptoms of food poisoning [77]. They can activate large populations of T-cells (~20–30%), resulting in a massive production of cytokines [78]. These protein toxins bind directly to major histocompatibility complex class II on antigen-presenting cells and specific Vβ regions of the T-cell receptor, leading to potentially life-threatening immune system stimulation [79]. This mechanism significantly contributes to the pathogenicity of *S. aureus* [79].

3. Conclusion

In conclusion, *S. aureus* demonstrates a wide range of virulence factors that significantly enhance its ability to cause disease. These factors enable the bacterium to efficiently colonize host tissues, evade immune responses, and cause substantial damage. By disrupting host cell membranes, manipulating coagulation pathways, and triggering excessive immune responses, *S. aureus* can persist and thrive within the host environment. Understanding these mechanisms highlights potential therapeutic targets and strategies for effectively managing and preventing *S. aureus* infections, emphasizing the importance of continued research in this field.

Acknowledgements

I would like to extend my sincere gratitude to the University of Jeddah for their support and resources that made this work possible.

Conflict of interest

The author declares no conflict of interest.

Author details

Dalal Alkuraythi
Department of Biology, College of Science, University of Jeddah, Jeddah,
Saudi Arabia

*Address all correspondence to: dalkrithi@uj.edu.sa

References

[1] Myles IA, Datta SK. *Staphylococcus aureus*: An introduction. Seminars in Immunopathology [Internet]. 2012;**34**(2):181-184. Available from: http://link.springer.com/10.1007/s00281-011-0301-9

[2] Tong SYC, Davis JS, Eichenberger E, Holland TL, Fowler VG. *Staphylococcus aureus* infections: Epidemiology, pathophysiology, clinical manifestations, and management. Clinical Microbiology Reviews [Internet]. 2015;**28**(3):603-661. Available from: http://cmr.asm.org/lookup/doi/10.1128/CMR.00134-14

[3] González-García S, Hamdan-Partida A, Bustos-Hamdan A, Bustos-Martínez J. Factors of nasopharynx that favor the colonization and persistence of *Staphylococcus aureus*. In: Pharynx - Diagnosis and Treatment. London, UK: IntechOpen; 2021

[4] Kwiecinski JM, Horswill AR. *Staphylococcus aureus* bloodstream infections: Pathogenesis and regulatory mechanisms. Current Opinion in Microbiology. 2020;**53**:51-60

[5] McGuinness WA, Malachowa N, DeLeo FR. Vancomycin resistance in *Staphylococcus aureus*. The Yale Journal of Biology and Medicine. 2017;**90**(2):269-281

[6] Chu VH, Crosslin DR, Friedman JY, Reed SD, Cabell CH, Griffiths RI, et al. *Staphylococcus aureus* bacteremia in patients with prosthetic devices: Costs and outcomes. The American Journal of Medicine [Internet]. 2005;**118**(12):1416.e19-1416.e24. Available from: https://linkinghub.elsevier.com/retrieve/pii/S0002934305004444

[7] McAdow M, Missiakas DM, Schneewind O. *Staphylococcus aureus* secretes coagulase and von Willebrand factor binding protein to modify the coagulation cascade and establish host infections. Journal of Innate Immunity [Internet]. 2012;**4**(2):141-148. Available from: https://www.karger.com/Article/FullText/333447

[8] Howden BP, Giulieri SG, Wong Fok Lung T, Baines SL, Sharkey LK, Lee JYH, et al. *Staphylococcus aureus* host interactions and adaptation. Nature Reviews Microbiology. 2023;**21**(6):380-395

[9] Jenul C, Horswill AR. Regulation of *Staphylococcus aureus* virulence. Gram-Positive Pathogens. 2019;**3**(12):948-958

[10] Novick RP. Autoinduction and signal transduction in the regulation of staphylococcal virulence. Molecular Microbiology [Internet]. 2003;**48**(6):1429-1449. Available from: http://doi.wiley.com/10.1046/j.1365-2958.2003.03526.x

[11] Wang X, Li X, Liu W, Huang W, Fu Q, Li M. Molecular characteristics and virulence gene profiles of community-associated methicillin-resistant *Staphylococcus aureus* isolates from pediatric patients in Shanghai, China. Frontiers in Microbiology. 2016;**7**:1818. DOI: 10.3389/fmicb.2016.01818

[12] Madani A, Garakani K, Mofrad MRK. Molecular mechanics of *Staphylococcus aureus* adhesin, CNA, and the inhibition of bacterial adhesion by stretching collagen. PLoS One [Internet]. 2017;**12**(6):e0179601. Available from: https://dx.plos.org/10.1371/journal.pone.0179601

[13] Paharik AE, Horswill AR. The staphylococcal biofilm: Adhesins, regulation, and host response.

Microbiology Spectrum. 2016;**4**(2). DOI: 10.1128/microbiolspec. VMBF-0022-2015

[14] Alorabi M, Ejaz U, Khoso B, Uddin F, Mahmoud S, Sohail M, et al. Detection of genes encoding microbial surface component recognizing adhesive matrix molecules in methicillin-resistant *Staphylococcus aureus* isolated from pyoderma patients. Genes (Basel). 2023;**14**(4):783

[15] Cheung GYC, Bae JS, Otto M. Pathogenicity and virulence of *Staphylococcus aureus*. Virulence. 2021;**12**(1):547-569

[16] Herman-Bausier P, Labate C, Towell AM, Derclaye S, Geoghegan JA, Dufrêne YF. *Staphylococcus aureus* clumping factor A is a force-sensitive molecular switch that activates bacterial adhesion. PNAS [Internet]. 2018;**115**(21):5564-5569. Available from: http://www.pnas.org/lookup/doi/10.1073/pnas.1718104115

[17] Wójcik-Bojek U, Różalska B, Sadowska B. *Staphylococcus aureus*—A known opponent against host defense mechanisms and vaccine development—Do we still have a chance to win? International Journal of Molecular Sciences. 2022;**23**(2):948

[18] Roche FM, Downer R, Keane F, Speziale P, Park PW, Foster TJ. The N-terminal a domain of fibronectin-binding proteins A and B promotes adhesion of *Staphylococcus aureus* to elastin. The Journal of Biological Chemistry [Internet]. 2004;**279**(37):38433-38440. Available from: http://www.jbc.org/lookup/doi/10.1074/jbc.M402122200

[19] Wu X, Wang H, Xiong J, Yang GX, Hu JF, Zhu Q, et al. *Staphylococcus aureus* biofilm: Formulation, regulatory, and emerging natural products-derived therapeutics. Biofilms. 2024;7:100175

[20] Herman-Bausier P, El-Kirat-Chatel S, Foster TJ, Geoghegan JA, Dufrêne YF. *Staphylococcus aureus* fibronectin-binding protein A mediates cell-cell adhesion through low-affinity homophilic bonds. mBio [Internet]. 2015;**6**(3). Available from: https://mbio.asm.org/lookup/doi/10.1128/mBio.00413-15

[21] Sharma S, Mohler J, Mahajan SD, Schwartz SA, Bruggemann L, Aalinkeel R. Microbial biofilm: A review on formation, infection, antibiotic resistance, control measures, and innovative treatment. Microorganisms. 2023;**11**(6):1614

[22] Foster TJ. The MSCRAMM family of cell-wall-anchored surface proteins of Gram-positive Cocci. Trends in Microbiology. 2019;**27**(11):927-941

[23] Piechota M, Kot B, Frankowska-Maciejewska A, Grużewska A, Woźniak-Kosek A. Biofilm formation by methicillin-resistant and methicillin-sensitive *Staphylococcus aureus* strains from hospitalized patients in Poland. BioMed Research International. 2018;**2018**:1-7

[24] Speziale P, Pietrocola G. The multivalent role of fibronectin-binding proteins A and B (FnBPA and FnBPB) of *Staphylococcus aureus* in host infections. Frontiers in Microbiology. 2020;**11**:2051. DOI: 10.3389/fmicb.2020.02051

[25] Park PW, Rosenbloom J, Abrams WR, Rosenbloom J, Mecham RP. Molecular cloning and expression of the gene for elastin-binding protein (ebpS) in *Staphylococcus aureus*. The Journal of Biological Chemistry [Internet]. 1996;**271**(26):15803-15809. Available from: http://www.jbc.org/lookup/doi/10.1074/jbc.271.26.15803

[26] Downer R, Roche F, Park PW, Mecham RP, Foster TJ. The

elastin-binding protein of *Staphylococcus aureus* (EbpS) is expressed at the cell surface as an integral membrane protein and not as a cell wall-associated protein. The Journal of Biological Chemistry. 2002;**277**(1):243-250

[27] Foster TJ. Surface proteins of *Staphylococcus aureus*. Microbiology Spectrum. 2019;**7**(4):1-16. DOI: 10.1128/microbiolspec.GPP3-0033-2018

[28] Ajayi C, Åberg E, Askarian F, Sollid JUE, Johannessen M, Hanssen AM. Genetic variability in the sdrD gene in *Staphylococcus aureus* from healthy nasal carriers. BMC Microbiology. 2018;**18**(1):34

[29] Harraghy N, Hussain M, Haggar A, Chavakis T, Sinha B, Herrmann M, et al. The adhesive and immunomodulating properties of the multifunctional *Staphylococcus aureus* protein Eap. Microbiology (NY) [Internet]. 2003;**149**(10):2701-2707. Available from: https://www.microbiologyresearch.org/content/journal/micro/10.1099/mic.0.26465-0

[30] Singh V, Phukan UJ. Interaction of host and *Staphylococcus aureus* protease-system regulates virulence and pathogenicity. Medical Microbiology and Immunology. 2019;**208**(5):585-607

[31] Nguyen HTT, Nguyen TH, Otto M. The staphylococcal exopolysaccharide PIA – Biosynthesis and role in biofilm formation, colonization, and infection. Computational and Structural Biotechnology Journal [Internet]. 2020;**18**:3324. Available from: https://pmc/articles/PMC7674160/ [Accessed: July 22, 2024]

[32] Nguyen LT, Vogel HJ. Staphylokinase has distinct modes of interaction with antimicrobial peptides, modulating its plasminogen-activation properties. Scientific Reports [Internet]. 2016;**6**. Available from: https://pmc/articles/PMC4995489/ [Accessed: July 22, 2024]

[33] Fattom A, Fuller S, Propst M, Winston S, Muenz L, He D, et al. Safety and immunogenicity of a booster dose of *Staphylococcus aureus* types 5 and 8 capsular polysaccharide conjugate vaccine (StaphVAX®) in hemodialysis patients. Vaccine [Internet]. 2004;**23**(5):656-663. Available from: https://linkinghub.elsevier.com/retrieve/pii/S0264410X04005341

[34] Cocchiaro JL, Gomez MI, Risley A, Solinga R, Sordelli DO, Lee JC. Molecular characterization of the capsule locus from non-typeable *Staphylococcus aureus*. Molecular Microbiology [Internet]. 2006;**59**(3):948-960. Available from: http://doi.wiley.com/10.1111/j.1365-2958.2005.04978.x

[35] Mohamed N, Timofeyeva Y, Jamrozy D, Rojas E, Hao L, Silmon de Monerri NC, et al. Molecular epidemiology and expression of capsular polysaccharides in *Staphylococcus aureus* clinical isolates in the United States. PLoS One [Internet]. 2019;**4**(1):e0208356. Available from: https://journals.plos.org/plosone/article?id=10.1371/journal.pone.0208356 [Accessed: July 22, 2024]

[36] Kuipers A, Stapels DAC, Weerwind LT, Ko YP, Ruyken M, Lee JC, et al. The *Staphylococcus aureus* polysaccharide capsule and Efb-dependent fibrinogen shield act in concert to protect against phagocytosis. Microbiology (NY) [Internet]. 2016;**162**(7):1185. Available from: https://pmc/articles/PMC4977062/ [Accessed: July 22, 2024]

[37] Yang B, Yao H, Li D, Liu Z. The phosphatidylglycerol phosphate synthase PgsA utilizes a trifurcated amphipathic cavity for catalysis at

the membrane-cytosol interface. Current Research in Structural Biology. 2021;**3**:312-323

[38] Tantawy E, Schwermann N, Ostermeier T, Garbe A, Bähre H, Vital M, et al. *Staphylococcus aureus* multiplexes death-effector deoxyribonucleosides to neutralize phagocytes. Frontiers in Immunology [Internet]. 2022;**13**:847171. Available from: www.frontiersin.org [Accessed: July 22, 2024]

[39] Thammavongsa V, Schneewind O, Missiakas DM. Enzymatic properties of *Staphylococcus aureus* adenosine synthase (AdsA). BMC Biochemistry [Internet]. 2011;**12**(1):56. Available from: https://pmc/articles/PMC3213008/ [Accessed: July 22, 2024]

[40] Postma B, Poppelier MJ, van Galen JC, Prossnitz ER, van Strijp JAG, de Haas CJC, et al. Chemotaxis inhibitory protein of *Staphylococcus aureus* binds specifically to the C5a and formylated peptide receptor. Journal of Immunology [Internet]. 2004;**172**(11):6994-7001. Available from: http://www.jimmunol.org/lookup/doi/10.4049/jimmunol.172.11.6994

[41] Sultan AR, Swierstra JW, Lemmens-den Toom NA, Snijders SV, Maňásková SH, Verbon A, et al. Production of staphylococcal complement inhibitor (SCIN) and other immune modulators during the early stages of *Staphylococcus aureus* biofilm formation in a mammalian cell culture medium. Infection and Immunity [Internet]. 2018;**86**(8). Available from: https://pmc/articles/PMC6056866/ [Accessed: July 23, 2024]

[42] Rooijakkers S, Milder F, Bardoel B, Ruyken M, van Roon J, Gros P, et al. Staphylococcal complement inhibitor (SCIN): Structure and active site. Molecular Immunology [Internet]. 2007;**44**(1-3):233. Available from: https://linkinghub.elsevier.com/retrieve/pii/S0161589006004354

[43] Jongerius I, Köhl J, Pandey MK, Ruyken M, Van Kessel KPM, Van Strijp JAG, et al. Staphylococcal complement evasion by various convertase-blocking molecules. The Journal of Experimental Medicine [Internet]. 2007;**204**(10):2461. Available from: https://pmc/articles/PMC2118443/ [Accessed: July 23, 2024]

[44] Atkins KL, Burman JD, Chamberlain ES, Cooper JE, Poutrel B, Bagby S, et al. *S. aureus* IgG-binding proteins SpA and Sbi: Host specificity and mechanisms of immune complex formation. Molecular Immunology [Internet]. 2008;**45**(6):1600-1611. Available from: https://linkinghub.elsevier.com/retrieve/pii/S0161589007007985

[45] Bear A, Locke T, Rowland-Jones S, Pecetta S, Bagnoli F, Darton TC. The immune evasion roles of *Staphylococcus aureus* protein A and impact on vaccine development. Frontiers in Cellular and Infection Microbiology [Internet]. 2023;**13**. Available from: https://pmc/articles/PMC10565657/ [Accessed: July 23, 2024]

[46] Kim HK, Emolo C, Missiakas D, Schneewind O. A monoclonal antibody that recognizes the E domain of staphylococcal protein A. Vaccine [Internet]. 2014;**32**(4):464. Available from: https://pmc/articles/PMC6211298/ [Accessed: July 23, 2024]

[47] Viela F, Prystopiuk V, Leprince A, Mahillon J, Speziale P, Pietrocola G, et al. Binding of *Staphylococcus aureus* protein A to von Willebrand factor is regulated by mechanical force. mBio [Internet]. 2019;**10**(2). Available from: https://pmc/articles/PMC6495375/ [Accessed: July 23, 2024]

[48] Burman J, Leung E, Isenman DE, van den Elsen JMH. Interaction of human complement with Sbi, a staphylococcal immunoglobulin-binding protein. Molecular Immunology [Internet]. 2007;**44**(16):3982. Available from: https://linkinghub.elsevier.com/retrieve/pii/S016158900700449X

[49] Dunphy RW, Wahid AA, Back CR, Martin RL, Watts AG, Dodson CA, et al. Staphylococcal complement evasion protein Sbi stabilises C3d dimers by inducing an N-terminal helix swap. Frontiers in Immunology [Internet]. 2022;**13**. Available from: https://pmc/articles/PMC9174452/ [Accessed: July 23, 2024]

[50] Hazmanian SK, Skaar EP, Gaspar AH, Humayun M, Gornicki P, Jelenska J, et al. Passage of heme-iron across the envelope of *Staphylococcus aureus*. Science [Internet]. 2003;**299**(5608):906-909. Available from: https://pubmed.ncbi.nlm.nih.gov/12574635/ [Accessed: July 23, 2024]

[51] Muryoi N, Tiedemann MT, Pluym M, Cheung J, Heinrichs DE, Stillman MJ. Demonstration of the iron-regulated surface determinant (Isd) heme transfer pathway in *Staphylococcus aureus*. The Journal of Biological Chemistry [Internet]. 2008;**283**(42):28125-28136. Available from: http://www.jbc.org/lookup/doi/10.1074/jbc.M802171200

[52] Sabat A, Kosowska K, Poulsen K, Kasprowicz A, Sekowska A, van den Burg B, et al. Two allelic forms of the aureolysin gene (*aur*) within *Staphylococcus aureus*. Infection and Immunity [Internet]. 2000;**68**(2):973-976. Available from: http://iai.asm.org/cgi/doi/10.1128/IAI.68.2.973-976.2000

[53] Tam K, Torres VJ. *Staphylococcus aureus* secreted toxins and extracellular enzymes. Microbiology Spectrum. 2019;**7**(2):1-20. DOI: 10.1128/microbiolspec.GPP3-0022-2018

[54] Makris G, Wright JD, Ingham E, Holland KT. The hyaluronate lyase of *Staphylococcus aureus* – A virulence factor? Microbiology (NY) [Internet]. 2004;**150**(6):2005-2013. Available from: https://www.microbiologyresearch.org/content/journal/micro/10.1099/mic.0.26942-0

[55] Hu C, Xiong N, Zhang Y, Rayner S, Chen S. Functional characterization of lipase in the pathogenesis of *Staphylococcus aureus*. Biochemical and Biophysical Research Communications [Internet]. 2012;**419**(4):617-620. Available from: https://linkinghub.elsevier.com/retrieve/pii/S0006291X12002902

[56] Hines KM, Alvarado G, Chen X, Gatto C, Pokorny A, Alonzo F, et al. Lipidomic and ultrastructural characterization of the cell envelope of *Staphylococcus aureus* grown in the presence of human serum. mSphere. 2020;**5**(3). DOI: 10.1128/mSphere.00357-20

[57] Demidyuk IV, Chukhontseva KN, Kostrov SV. Glutamyl endopeptidases: The puzzle of substrate specificity. Acta Naturae. 2017;**9**(2):17-33

[58] Karlsson A, Arvidson S. Variation in extracellular protease production among clinical isolates of *Staphylococcus aureus* due to different levels of expression of the protease repressor sarA. Infection and Immunity. 2002;**70**(8):4239-4246

[59] Frey AM, Chaput D, Shaw LN. Insight into the human pathodegradome of the V8 protease from *Staphylococcus aureus*. Cell Reports. 2021;**35**(1):108930

[60] Pietrocola G, Nobile G, Rindi S, Speziale P. *Staphylococcus aureus* manipulates innate immunity through

own and host-expressed proteases. Frontiers in Cellular and Infection Microbiology. 2017;**7**:166

[61] Kantyka T, Pyrc K, Gruca M, Smagur J, Plaza K, Guzik K, et al. *Staphylococcus aureus* proteases degrade lung surfactant protein A potentially impairing innate immunity of the lung. Journal of Innate Immunity. 2013;**5**(3):251-260

[62] Thomas S, Liu W, Arora S, Ganesh V, Ko YP, Höök M. The complex fibrinogen interactions of the *Staphylococcus aureus* coagulases. Frontiers in Cellular and Infection Microbiology. 2019;**9**:20. DOI: 10.3389/fcimb.2019.00020

[63] Nappi F, Avtaar Singh SS. Host–bacterium interaction mechanisms in *Staphylococcus aureus* endocarditis: A systematic review. International Journal of Molecular Sciences. 2023;**24**(13):11068

[64] Cruz AR, van Strijp JAG, Bagnoli F, Manetti AGO. Virulence gene expression of *Staphylococcus aureus* in human skin. Frontiers in Microbiology. 2021;**12**:649323. DOI: 10.3389/fmicb.2021.649323

[65] Unnikrishnan M, Constantinidou C, Palmer T, Pallen MJ. The enigmatic Esx proteins: Looking beyond mycobacteria. Trends in Microbiology [Internet]. 2017;**25**(3):192-204. Available from: https://linkinghub.elsevier.com/retrieve/pii/S0966842X16301676

[66] Kengmo Tchoupa A, Watkins KE, Jones RA, Kuroki A, Alam MT, Perrier S, et al. The type VII secretion system protects *Staphylococcus aureus* against antimicrobial host fatty acids. Scientific Reports. 2020;**10**(1):14838

[67] Kaneko J, Kamio Y. Bacterial two-component and hetero-heptameric pore-forming cytolytic toxins: Structures, pore-forming mechanism, and organization of the genes. Bioscience, Biotechnology, and Biochemistry. 2004;**68**(5):981-1003

[68] Inoshima I, Inoshima N, Wilke GA, Powers ME, Frank KM, Wang Y, et al. A *Staphylococcus aureus* pore-forming toxin subverts the activity of ADAM10 to cause lethal infection in mice. Nature Medicine [Internet]. 2011;**17**(10):1310-1314. Available from: http://www.nature.com/articles/nm.2451

[69] Zhu Z, Hu Z, Li S, Fang R, Ono HK, Hu DL. Molecular characteristics and pathogenicity of *Staphylococcus aureus* exotoxins. International Journal of Molecular Sciences. 2023;**25**(1):395

[70] Vandenesch F, Lina G, Henry T. *Staphylococcus aureus* hemolysins, bi-component leukocidins, and cytolytic peptides: A redundant arsenal of membrane-damaging virulence factors? Frontiers in Cellular and Infection Microbiology. 2012;**2**:12. DOI: 10.3389/fcimb.2012.00012

[71] Oliveira D, Borges A, Simões M. *Staphylococcus aureus* toxins and their molecular activity in infectious diseases. Toxins (Basel). 2018;**10**(6):252

[72] Bouillot S, Reboud E, Huber P. Functional consequences of calcium influx promoted by bacterial pore-forming toxins. Toxins (Basel). 2018;**10**(10):387

[73] Bukowski M, Wladyka B, Dubin G. Exfoliative toxins of *Staphylococcus aureus*. Toxins (Basel). 2010;**2**(5):1148-1165

[74] Plano LRW. *Staphylococcus aureus* exfoliative toxins: How they cause disease. Journal of Investigative Dermatology. 2004;**122**(5):1070-1077

[75] Zarei Koosha R, Mahmoodzadeh Hosseini H, Mehdizadeh Aghdam E, Ghorbani Tajandareh S, Imani Fooladi AA. Distribution of *tsst*-1 and *mec*A genes in *Staphylococcus aureus* isolated from clinical specimens. Jundishapur Journal of Microbiology [Internet]. 2016;**9**(3). Available from: http://jjmicrobiol.neoscriber.org/en/articles/56605.html

[76] Deacy AM, Gan SKE, Derrick JP. Superantigen recognition and interactions: Functions, mechanisms and applications. Frontiers in Immunology. 2021;**12**:731211. DOI: 10.3389/fimmu.2021.731211

[77] Argudín MÁ, Mendoza MC, Rodicio MR. Food poisoning and *Staphylococcus aureus* enterotoxins. Toxins (Basel). 2010;**2**(7):1751-1773

[78] Pinchuk IV, Beswick EJ, Reyes VE. Staphylococcal enterotoxins. Toxins (Basel). 2010;**2**(8):2177-2197

[79] Krakauer T. Staphylococcal superantigens: Pyrogenic toxins induce toxic shock. Toxins (Basel). 2019;**11**(3):178

Chapter 2

Staphylococcus aureus Biofilms: Characteristics and Impacts on the Treatment of Infectious Diseases

Nara Juliana Santos Araújo, Vanessa Lima Bezerra,
Maria do Socorro Costa, Camila Aparecida Pereira da Silva,
Ana Raquel Pereira da Silva, Damiana Gonçalves de Sousa Freitas,
Josefa Sayonara dos Santos, Juliete Bezerra Soares
and Jacqueline Cosmo Andrade-Pinheiro

Abstract

Bacterial biofilms have been the subject of studies, mainly because they are responsible for a significant fraction of persistent infections that are resistant to both the action of antimicrobials and the action of the host's immune system. *Staphylococcus aureus* is a pathogen with remarkable virulence, present in a significant portion of infectious diseases that affect humans, and its ability to form biofilms contributes to the risks associated with outbreaks involving this agent. This chapter aims to highlight and understand the molecular components involved in the formation and maturation of *S. aureus* biofilms, as well as the host's immune responses. These factors are crucial for developing effective strategies to overcome the resistance barrier imposed by biofilms, with the goal of implementing more effective treatments and improving patients' quality of life. Additionally, the chapter will address the current therapies available for treating infections caused by *S. aureus* biofilms.

Keywords: *Staphylococcus aureus*, biofilms, infection, resistance, treatment

1. Introduction

Staphylococcus aureus is widely recognized as one of the main etiological agents causing several hospital infections and diseases, such as endocarditis, osteomyelitis, bacteremia, pneumonia, skin infections, and complications associated with implanted devices [1].

Biofilm formation is a crucial virulence factor that influences the pathogenicity of the genus *Staphylococcus* in infections related mainly to devices. Biofilms are defined

IntechOpen

as microbial communities adhered to surfaces, encapsulated by an extracellular polymeric matrix that offers protection against the host immune system and conventional antimicrobial treatments [2].

Staphylococcus aureus biofilms represent one of the greatest challenges in the treatment of infectious diseases, resulting in an incidence of the infectious process in approximately 80% of cases, especially when it comes to infections occurring within intensive care units [3]. Its ability to form biofilms is associated with chronic infections, which contributes to resistance to conventional therapies. Studies focused on the molecular components involved in the process of biofilm formation and maturation are important for the development of strategies that contribute to reversing resistance and ensuring effective treatments, improving patients' quality of life [4, 5].

It is well known that the formation of biofilms in *Staphylococcus aureus* contributes significantly to the development of resistance to conventional antibiotics, biocides, and even the host's natural defenses, in addition to promoting the production of several virulence factors [1, 2]. In view of this clinical emergency, the need to explore new alternatives in the development of effective drugs against biofilm-associated diseases has become an urgent priority in modern medicine. Continued research and advancement of innovative therapeutic strategies are crucial to combating this growing public health threat.

This study aims to analyze the molecular mechanisms involved in the formation and maturation of *Staphylococcus aureus* biofilms and how these mechanisms contribute to resistance to antimicrobial treatments. Additionally, it aims to explore host immune responses and evaluate both current and emerging therapies for the control and treatment of biofilm-associated infections. Understanding these aspects is essential for developing more effective and innovative therapeutic strategies that can improve infection management and patient's quality of life.

2. Characteristics of *Staphylococcus aureus* biofilms

2.1 Composition and structure of biofilms

Staphylococcus aureus presents two main structures in biofilm formation: the extracellular matrix and microcolonies. Several characteristics of biofilms, such as increased resistance to antibiotics, adaptability, and strong adhesion to surfaces, are closely related to the extracellular matrix secreted by this microorganism. This matrix, of viscous consistency, represents about 90% of the dry mass of the biofilm and is composed of polymeric substances, extracellular DNA (eDNA), proteins, and polysaccharides [2, 6].

Unlike other microorganisms that possess several exopolysaccharides (EPS), *Staphylococci* produce only one dominant EPS molecule, the polysaccharide intercellular adhesin (PIA) or poly-β (1–6)-N-acetylglucosamine (PNAG) which is the agent of intercellular adhesion and adhesion to external surfaces [5, 7, 8].

The cell surface of *S. aureus* is composed of more than 20 proteins covalently anchored to peptidoglycan by the enzyme sortase A. These proteins, known as cell wall proteins (CWA), can be classified into different groups based on their structural and functional characteristics [7, 9]. Some examples include Clumping factor A (ClfA) and Clumping factor B (ClfB), which bind to fibrinogen and facilitate the formation of biofilms. Additionally, fibronectin-binding proteins (FnBPs), such as FnbA and FnbB, interact with fibronectin, while Collagen-binding protein (Can) binds to collagen. Serine-aspartate repeat proteins C, D, and E (SdrC, SdrD, and SdrE) also play a role in adhesion and colonization, along with other families of proteins related to bacterial survival [9].

Another important component of the biofilm structure is the extracellular DNA (eDNA) molecules, which are present in the matrix and are released after cell death. *S. aureus* biofilms show variations in eDNA content between different strains, and these variations are significantly affected by environmental conditions, including antibiotic exposure. It facilitates the process of irreversible attachment, phenazine retention, and contributes to the process of bacterial resistance [5, 10–13].

The structural process of biofilm formation by *S. aureus* involves several steps. This structure is established by the attachment of bacterial cells to the surface, followed by the formation of microcolonies. As the microcolonies consolidate, synthesis of the extracellular matrix that provides structural support begins. Biofilms are organized in layers that allow the diffusion of nutrients. In this environment, cells can undergo aerobic growth, fermentation, death, or dormancy [2, 14, 15].

2.2 Mechanisms of biofilm formation

Biofilm formation by *S. aureus* occurs through the stages of attachment (adhesion to the surface), aggregation (accumulation and multiplication), maturation (mature biofilm), and dispersion (final phase of the biofilm life cycle). One of the crucial stages is the attachment of planktonic cells to the surface which occurs due to hydrophilic and hydrophobic interactions between the bacterial cell and the target surface mediated by adhesion proteins present on the bacterial cell surface. However, this initial stage of formation is potentially reversible [2, 16, 17].

During the initial stage, planktonic cells of *S. aureus* use different factors and mechanisms, such as adhesins, alteration of the bacterial cell surface, and the production of eDNA to interact with the host, through proteins anchored in the cell wall. In addition to these factors, the autolytic enzymes AtlA are the main facilitators for primary attachment to surfaces [4, 5].

After the adhesion process, cell multiplication begins and the cell is incorporated into the matrix, which is composed of a complex set of extracellular polymeric substances, such as polysaccharides, proteins, lipids, extracellular DNA, and other biomolecules. It has a rigid and thick structure [16–19].

The last stage is cell dispersal, in which the *quorum sensing* system, which regulates the behavior of bacteria within the biofilm, releases chemical signals that promote separation and dispersal, allowing the bacterial cells to return to the planktonic state [20].

2.3 Environmental and biological conditions for *Staphylococcus aureus* biofilm formation

Three main factors contribute to the formation of *Staphylococcus* biofilm: the ability to adhere to surfaces, the host immune response, and environmental factors [21].

The ability to adhere to these devices occurs through two main pathways. The first occurs through direct interaction with the surface, while the second involves the formation of connections with proteins in the extracellular matrix. In general, biofilms tend to form where nutrients such as carbon, nitrogen, and phosphate are abundant and can begin to dissolve when nutrients are depleted [15, 22, 23].

Biofilms increase the ability of bacteria to survive environmental stresses, in addition to being potential reservoirs of pathogens such as *S. aureus* [24]. However, factors such as pH, temperature, nutrient availability, salinity, and dissolved oxygen play crucial roles in the development and persistence of *Staphylococcus* biofilms. According to recent studies, the biofilm formation capacity of *S. aureus* is optimal at temperatures between 25°C and 37°C, while lower temperatures, such as 10°C and 4°C, significantly reduce this capacity. Furthermore, the addition of NaCl has been shown to further favor biofilm formation [25].

3. Impacts of *Staphylococcus aureus* biofilms on the treatment of infectious diseases

3.1 Resistance to antibiotics

The biofilm acts as a shield against environmental conditions that are unfavorable to the survival of the bacteria, protecting it from the action of the host's immune system and restricting the penetration and damage caused by drugs. This shield plays a fundamental role in the development of antimicrobial resistance and therapeutic failure, especially in the case of strains of *Staphylococcus aureus* [16, 26].

The main characteristics responsible for the resistance presented by biofilms include the limited diffusion of antimicrobial agents through the biofilm matrix, the communication of antimicrobial agents with the biofilm matrix, enzyme-mediated resistance, the levels of metabolic activity within the biofilm, genetic adaptation, efflux pumps, and the structure of the outer membrane. The matrix has an efflux system and enzymes that are capable of inactivating antimicrobials and protecting the peripheral region of the biofilm [27, 28].

Staphylococcus aureus infections associated with biofilms do not respond positively to treatment, even when administering antibiotics that show effective results when tested in standard susceptibility tests since the tests used in clinical laboratories to analyze the susceptibility of microorganisms in relation to antibiotics do not cover the behavior of *S. aureus* associated with biofilms, as they are performed on planktonic bacteria [29, 30].

The *Quorum sensing* system, in addition to its functions in the formation and intercellular communication in the biofilm, also plays important roles in virulence and antimicrobial resistance in *S. aureus*. In this species, this system is also called the accessory gene regulator (*agr*), encoded by the *agr locus* [31]. The *Agr* system also regulates the detachment of biofilm cells from the matrix, and these can cause systemic infections or even adhere to another location and form a new biofilm [32].

The S. *aureus* bacteria present in the biofilm can alter their gene expression in response to antibiotics such as ampicillin, leading to the translation of genes encoding antimicrobial resistance mechanisms. These include genes for the AbcA efflux pump, modified penicillin-binding proteins (PBP1a/2), and antimicrobial resistance protein genes such as VraF, VraG, Dlt, and Aur. Furthermore, the expression of genes encoding surface proteins such as clumping factor B (ClfB), iron-regulated surface determinant (IsdA), and *S. aureus* surface protein (SasG), as well as genes that promote adhesion (cap5B and cap5C) induced by ampicillin, increases biofilm viability and biomass [33, 34].

Polysaccharide intercellular adhesin (PIA) is the only exopolysaccharide in *Staphylococcus aureus* and, in addition to its function in biofilm formation and evasion of the host immune system, it also plays a role in the virulence and antibacterial resistance of the species. This molecule, which is part of the extracellular matrix, mainly affects the penetration of antibiotics into the biofilm, but it can also, in some way, limit the activity of antibiotics that have no difficulty in overcoming the matrix barrier [8].

Another important factor in bacterial resistance is the two-component system encoded by the yycFG gene, which consists of the regulatory protein (YycF) and the sensory protein (YycG). This system is responsible for the generation of *Staphylococcus aureus* strains with intermediate resistance to vancomycin (VISA) and *Staphylococcus aureus* with heteroresistance to vancomycin (hVISA). This gene also confers resistance to depolarization and/or permeabilization, contributing to resistance to daptomycin and many other resistance mechanisms, such as the metabolism of cell wall peptidoglycans, the metabolism of cell membrane lipids, and evasion of the innate immune system, are directly or indirectly regulated by it [35, 36].

Antibiotic resistance is reinforced by a transition of the colony from an exponentially multiplying state to a slowly multiplying or non-multiplying state. When antibiotics are administered, they kill most of the cells and the immune system kills both the regular cells and the persister cells in the bloodstream, but some persister cells remain in the biofilm [37].

The biofilm community has a high cell density, which can cause an uneven distribution of nutrients and oxygen, which deprives some cells of this supply. Because of this, the cells reduce their metabolic activity and energy status, a state called persistence, and can survive exposure to most bactericidal antibiotics. In addition, an antibiotic concentration gradient is generated, resulting in selective pressure for these cells to change their state to a persistence state, due to the presence of sub-inhibitory concentrations of this drug [38].

These persistent cells, or persisters, are a specific subpopulation of cells capable of developing temporary antibiotic resistance phenotypes, since these cells are in a metabolic state of dormancy, not undergoing cell division. Since antibiotics require active targets to exert their effect and kill the bacterial cell, when an antibiotic is administered to a population, the metabolically active cells die, while the persisters survive and, in the absence of the antibiotic, repopulate the biofilm, and the infection returns. From this, it is possible to suggest that these cells may be the primary contributors to the recurrence of chronic infections resistant to antimicrobial therapy [7, 39].

In *S. aureus*, there is an eventual shift to a stationary phase in metabolism, generating a decrease in intracellular ATP. The low concentration of ATP is one of the causes of the tolerance of this microorganism to antimicrobials and represents a lower probability of therapeutic efficacy. These cells may be present throughout the growth phase, but increase proportionally to the increase in cell density in the biofilm [5, 40].

Since persister cells are dormant and are not susceptible to antibiotics available in the clinic, biotechnological approaches have been developed to combat these dormant cells, using compounds that are capable of entering the cell without active transport and can kill the cells without the need for any cellular metabolism mechanism [37].

3.2 Immune response to biofilm infection

The immune system responds to biofilm infection, but unlike the action against planktonic cells, the immune response is quite ineffective most of the time and can lead to recalcitrant infections and even chronic infection [41]. This is mainly due to the physical and mechanical properties of these biofilms, which allow them to evade immune cells, including allowing them to resist elimination by phagocytosis. The entire metabolome of the biofilm is modified when it encounters the host's defense cells, even leading to an increase in damage to the host generated by the inflammatory response itself [42, 43].

Neutrophils, the first line of defense against bacteria, can invade the biofilm structure, but the community can reverse the attack by producing *quorum sensing*-regulated toxins that inhibit immune recognition and activity. In addition, the biofilm can produce detergent-like molecules that have direct cytotoxic activity against these cells [41].

This inflammatory response occurs early and is ineffective, mainly due to the fact that complement fixation occurs, to which *S. aureus* and other Gram-positive species are essentially resistant. And, it is this early response that triggers the activation of neutrophils and the release of inflammatory mediators that cause tissue damage, are harmful to the host, and some mediators, such as IL-1β, can even reinforce biofilm formation [44].

The persistence, dissemination, or elimination of infection is determined by the interaction between *S. aureus* and macrophages, because as the infection persists, macrophages switch to an anti-inflammatory phenotype. *S. aureus* biofilm increases the challenges in eliminating the bacteria by avoiding recognition by macrophages, tolerating phagocytosis, reprogramming the metabolic patterns of host cells, promoting anti-inflammatory polarization, and inducing cell death [45].

In a chronic response, the host produces IgG-class antibodies to combat the infection. However, due to heterogeneity within the biofilm community, an antigen may be produced in some areas and not in others, leading to ineffective antigen recognition by antibodies and a failure to eliminate these microorganisms [44]. In this way, the biofilm allows bacteria, especially strains of *S. aureus*, a multicellular strategy that reverses the relationship between the host's immune cells and the pathogen [46].

3.3 Complications in clinical treatment resulting from the presence of biofilm

Staphylococcus aureus species are among the first biofilm-forming strains recorded on hospital devices, being commonly related to cases of septicemia, especially in patients with burns and implanted medical devices, whether temporary or permanent [47]. Device or wound infections are associated with opportunistic organisms such as *Staphylococcus aureus* and are difficult to treat, requiring debridement and even removal of the device, depending on the severity, in addition to presenting a high morbidity and mortality rate [48]. Such infections are observed in a considerable number of patients, being more frequent in immunocompromised individuals [49].

The presence of biofilm makes it difficult to treat pathologies because it can inhibit the penetration of antibiotics so that they can act, in addition to being capable of inactivating them through enzymatic decomposition or adsorption, resulting in relapses or complications [50]. In *Staphylococcus aureus* strains, the presence of biofilm can generate an increase in antibiotic resistance in the range of 10–1000 times, in addition to contributing to the dissemination of the genes responsible for such resistance, making the healing process difficult [51], requiring high doses of antimicrobials which, often, can lead to an increase in the systemic toxicity of the drugs [52], with high rates of mortality, relapse, and treatment failures having been observed [23].

Antimicrobial resistance may be related to phenomena such as the anaerobic metabolism of bacteria, enzyme production, and the presence of the matrix that acts as an efficient physical barrier that can prevent the entry or dispersion of antimicrobials, hindering their action and causing complications in treatment, requiring the need for more extreme interventions such as surgical procedures [53, 54].

3.4 *Staphylococcus aureus* biofilm in the nosocomial environment

Bacterial biofilm can be observed in clinical conditions such as infective endocarditis, where it disrupts valve function [55], sepsis [56], and osteomyelitis [57]. The presence of this bacterial organization directly contributes to the increased morbidity and mortality of patients with such pathologies [56]. The presence of biofilm can lead to the inefficiency of antimicrobials, leading to inadequate treatment that can result in recurrence in approximately 80% of cases [3].

When it comes to infections occurring within intensive care units, cases of *Staphylococcus aureus* detection are the second most recorded type, with 10 cases recorded for every 1000 patients using mechanical ventilators and approximately 3.9 cases for every 1000 patients using central catheters and indwelling catheters [58, 59].

The scientific literature classifies the presence of biofilms as a relevant factor of clinical complication, however, it reports the scarcity of studies on this topic and the importance of carrying out more in-depth studies, considering that many deals with detection and eradication and not exclusively with their nosocomial impact [60], which demonstrates the importance of determining factors such as epidemiological, molecular, phenotypic, and pathophysiological aspects of such infections [61].

In addition to developing profiles related to microorganisms and the structure of the biofilm, it is necessary to implement hygiene, disinfection, and antimicrobial exposure processes in order to prevent the transmission of infectious agents in the nosocomial environment [58].

4. New therapeutic approaches to combat *Staphylococcus aureus* biofilms

Biofilm production leads to a significant increase in drug resistance of *Staphylococcus aureus*, demanding the need for new therapies to combat it. Among these, enzyme therapy has been a treatment option due to its potential to disrupt the bacterial matrix [18, 62, 63]. The action of these enzymes, such as glycoside hydrolases and proteases, is directly related to the molecular complexity of the biofilm and the characteristics of the substrate [64, 65]. Its enhancement can be obtained through the mixture of different enzymes, which has shown more effective action, compared to the use of isolated enzymes [66].

Biofilm control by phages emerges as a new paradigm for possible therapies against *S. aureus.* In addition to phages, proteins synthesized by phages have been widely studied and have shown potential antibacterial agents. Enzymes, such as virion-associated peptidoglycan hydrolases (VAPGHs), endolysins, and depolymerases, are used by phages to interact with and kill hosts [67, 68].

Nanostructures increase the therapeutic efficacy of many drugs by enhancing their efficiency and bioavailability. They also support significant advances in the selectivity of drug-receptor interactions, systemic bioavailability, and controlled drug release. This is exemplified by polymeric nanoparticles, which are more effective in combating bacteria than the free antimicrobial agents themselves [69].

Nanoparticles have diverse applications in multiple areas of modern science [70]. Some studies have presented polypyrrole nanoparticles and phytofabricated metal nanoparticles as a substantial option against *S. aureus*, as well as silver nanoparticles associated with simvastatin and copper complexes derived from Schiff base combined with oxacillin and vancomycin as potential promising antimicrobial and antibiofilm agents in the fight against infections originating from *S. aureus* [71–74].

Essential oils combined with different antibiotics have shown good results in destroying biofilms, probably due to the presence of monoterpenes, phenols, and alcohols in their composition [75, 76]. The combination of traditional antibiotics, such as norfloxacin, oxacillin, and gentamicin, with certain essential oils, such as *Cinnamomum zeylanicum*, *Mentha piperita*, *Origanum vulgare*, and *Thymus vulgaris*, has shown potent activity against *Staphylococcus aureus* biofilms. This association may be a beginning for the creation of safer drug formulations [76].

4.1 Emerging technologies and development of antibiofilm materials

Among the most promising approaches, antibiofilm coatings stand out, which mainly aim to prevent the initial adhesion of bacteria to surfaces. In this context, coating nanoengineering falls into this category, as it aims to alter the physicochemical characteristics of substrate surfaces in such a way that interactions with surfaces and bacteria become unfavorable [77].

The creation of low-adhesion surfaces has proven to be a promising technique for the non-toxic control of microbial bioadhesion. Several approaches have been used, such as topographic modifications, which are designed to destabilize biofilms and reduce irreversible attachment, developing selective anti-fouling effects on certain species [78, 79]. Furthermore, the use of antimicrobial substances, such as antibiotics [79, 80], antimicrobial peptides [81, 82], and quaternary ammonium compounds, have been shown to be effective when applied as special coatings to prevent biofilm formation [81, 83, 84].

The use of polymers, in turn, stands out as a widely used approach for non-stick surfaces, using several mechanisms to prevent bacterial adhesion. Among the polymeric strategies, steric hydration is the most investigated, as it forms a layer of strongly associated water, which reduces the contact angle with water and gives these surfaces a superhydrophilic characteristic [85].

In addition to the use of polymers, recent research has explored nature-inspired surfaces to prevent bacterial adhesion [86], such as plant leaves [87], dragonfly wings, cicada wings [88], lizard skin [89], and shark skin [90]. These bio-inspired architectures are replicated by surface engineering due to their anti-fouling and antibacterial properties, being used in the development of synthetic antimicrobial surfaces through nanoscience tools [91, 92].

Photodynamic therapy, which combines visible light, a photosensitizer, and oxygen to induce a phototoxic reaction capable of killing bacteria, has shown promise. Photosensitizers, when exposed to a specific wavelength of light, generate free radicals and reactive oxygen species that cause oxidative damage to bacteria, affecting essential molecules such as DNA, RNA, proteins, and lipids. Due to the distributed nature of this damage, photodynamic therapy has been considered the least likely to promote the development of antimicrobial resistance [93, 94].

Finally, *quorum sensing* inhibition has emerged as a promising strategy to prevent the synthesis of factors that contribute to biofilm formation. One example is apicidin, a fungal metabolite that acts as an inhibitor in *quorum sensing* communication [95]. In recent decades, interference in bacterial communication has become an intensely explored field of research. This approach seeks to identify molecules that act specifically on the quorum sensing system, reducing the production of exoenzymes and toxins without interfering with bacterial growth, qualifying as an ideal adjuvant therapy that can be combined with antibiotics to increase the efficacy of antimicrobial therapy and decrease the risk of resistance [4].

4.2 Prevention and control of *Staphylococcus aureus* biofilms in clinical settings

The application of effective hygiene and sterilization protocols is crucial to prevent infections in clinical settings, especially those caused by *Staphylococcus aureus* biofilms, which are highly resistant to conventional treatments. Given this resistance, it is essential to implement rigorous and updated control strategies to minimize the risks associated with these infections [96].

Adopting hygienic and sanitary practices and sanitation procedures is essential to prevent the development of infections. These measures include rigorous hand washing, disinfection of materials used, and training staff to recognize the risks of transmission caused by multidrug-resistant bacteria. In environments with a high probability of transmission and development of resistant microorganisms, defining well-structured hygiene and sterilization protocols is essential [97].

In the context of sterilization protocols, the use of autoclaves is widely adopted, as they employ heat and pressure to kill microorganisms and their spores. However, some devices used in clinical settings are heat-sensitive, which necessitates the adoption of alternative sterilization methods [98].

Hydrogen peroxide sterilization, in turn, is widely used due to its compatibility with most medical devices, as well as its proven efficacy and safety [99]. Although ethylene oxide gas sterilization has been considered the gold standard due to its effectiveness, it has significant disadvantages, such as long processing times and the generation of toxic and carcinogenic residues [98].

In addition to these methods, the use of ultrasound for biofilm removal has gained prominence, especially in clinical settings, due to its effectiveness and potential to complement traditional disinfection and cleaning methods. Ultrasound utilizes high-frequency sound waves to generate cavitations, which are the formation of cavities that can destabilize biofilms and even inactivate microorganisms [100]. Other physical methods, such as plasma application, have also been employed in biofilm eradication. Plasma offers advantages over traditional methods, as it contains free radicals, charged particles, electrons, photons, and other particles that can effectively interact to destroy biofilms [100, 101].

Despite the adoption of several disinfection procedures in healthcare settings, the presence of biofilms in these settings suggests that cleaning and disinfection protocols may be insufficient. Although biofilms contribute to failures in prevention and disinfection, they are not the only culprits. To address these challenges, it is essential to train healthcare professionals to recognize the risks associated with biofilms and implement effective measures to prevent contamination and infections [102].

5. Conclusion

The biofilm acts as a shield that protects *Staphylococcus aureus* against mechanical actions, immune response, and antimicrobial action. This structure is frequently associated with nosocomial infections and is considered a relevant cause of complications and morbidity and mortality in patients, especially those who are immunocompromised, increasing hospitalization periods and therefore requiring the need for more in-depth studies that can provide elimination and prevention profiles to ensure a better prognosis for patients. Several lines of research have gained prominence in the fight against biofilms, some examples being innovative therapeutic approaches, such as the use of enzymes, combination therapies, and others, which offer new perspectives in the fight against *Staphylococcus aureus* biofilms. Although promising, these strategies still face challenges for their effective clinical application. The integration of these techniques with rigorous hygiene and sterilization protocols is essential to overcome current limitations and achieve effective control of these resistant infections.

Acknowledgements

To the Laboratory of Microbiology and Molecular Biology—LMBM, Regional University of Cariri (URCA) Brazil; the Laboratory of Applied Microbiology—LAMAP, Federal University of Cariri©UFCA, to the National Council for Scientific and Technological Development—CNPq, to the Coordination Foundation for the Improvement of Higher Education Personnel—CAPES, and to the Ceará Foundation for the Support of Scientific and Technological Development—FUNCAP, for financing the project Susceptibility of Bacterial Biofilms to Steroidal Sapogenins (#BP5-0197 00189.01.00/22).

Conflict of interest

The authors declare no conflict of interest.

Author details

Nara Juliana Santos Araújo[1,2,5], Vanessa Lima Bezerra[1,2,5], Maria do Socorro Costa[1,3,5], Camila Aparecida Pereira da Silva[1,3,5], Ana Raquel Pereira da Silva[1], Damiana Gonçalves de Sousa Freitas[1,4], Josefa Sayonara dos Santos[1,5], Juliete Bezerra Soares[1,5] and Jacqueline Cosmo Andrade-Pinheiro[1,2,3,5]*

1 Laboratory of Applied Microbiology—LAMAP, Federal University of Cariri, Barbalha, Ceará, Brazil

2 Multicenter Postgraduate Program in Biochemistry and Molecular Biology, Federal University of Cariri, Barbalha, Ceará, Brazil

3 Postgraduate Program in Health Sciences, Federal University of Cariri, Barbalha, Ceará, Brazil

4 Regional University of Cariri—URCA, Crato, Ceará, Brazil

5 Federal University of Cariri—UFCA, Crato, Ceará, Brazil

*Address all correspondence to: jaqueline.andrade@ufca.edu.br

References

[1] Parai D, Banerjee M, Dey P, Mukherjee SK. Reserpine attenuates biofilm formation and virulence of *Staphylococcus aureus*. Microbial Pathogenesis. 2020;**138**:103790. DOI: 10.1016/j.micpath.2019.103790

[2] Idrees M, Sawant S, Karodia N, Rahman A. *Staphylococcus aureus* biofilm: Morphology, genetics, pathogenesis and treatment strategies. International Journal of Environmental Research and Public Health. 2021;**18**:7602. DOI: 10.3390/ijerph18147602

[3] Tuon FF, Suss PH, Telles JP, Dantas LR, Borges NH, Ribeiro VST. Antimicrobial treatment of *Staphylococcus aureus* biofilms. Antibiotics. 2023;**12**:1-24. DOI: 10.3390/antibiotics12010087

[4] Schilcher K, Horswill AR. *Staphylococcal* biofilm development: Structure, regulation, and treatment strategies. Microbiology and Molecular Biology Reviews. 2020;**84**(3):10-1128. DOI: 10.1128/mmbr.00026-19

[5] Guo H, Tong Y, Cheng J, Abbas Z, Li Z, Wang J, et al. Biofilm and small colony variants—An update on *Staphylococcus aureus* strategies toward drug resistance. International Journal of Molecular Sciences. 2022;**23**:1241. DOI: 10.3390/ijms23031241

[6] Hiltunen AK, Savijoki K, Nyman TA, Miettinen I, Ihalainen P, Peltonen J, et al. Structural and functional dynamics of *Staphylococcus aureus* biofilms and biofilm matrix proteins on different clinical materials. Microorganisms. 2019;**7**:584. DOI: 10.3390/microorganisms7120584

[7] Parastan R, Kargar M, Solhjoo K, Kafilzadeh F. *Staphylococcus aureus* biofilms: Structures, antibiotic resistance, inhibition, and vacines. Gene Reports. 2020;**20**:1-8. DOI: 10.1016/j.genrep.2020.100739

[8] Nguyen HTT, Nguyen TH, Otto M. The staphylococcal exopolysaccharide PIA – Biosynthesis and role in biofilm formation, colonization, and infection. Computational and Structural Biotechnology Journal. 2020;**18**:3324-3334. DOI: 10.1016/j.csbj.2020.10.027

[9] Foster TJ. Surface proteins of *Staphylococcus aureus*. Microbiology Spectrum. 2019;**7**:1-22. DOI: 10.1128/microbiolspec.gpp3-0046-2018

[10] Bowden LC, Finlinson J, Jones B, Berges BK. Beyond the double helix: The multifaceted landscape of extracellular DNA in *Staphylococcus aureus* biofilms. Frontiers in Cellular and Infection Microbiology. 2024;**14**:1-13. DOI: 10.3389/fcimb.2024.1400648

[11] Mann EE, Arroz KC, Boles BR, Endres JL, Ranjit D, Chandramohan L, et al. Modulation of eDNA release and degradation affects *Staphylococcus aureus* biofilm maturation. PLoS One. 2009;**4**:1-12. DOI: 10.1371/journal.pone.0005822

[12] Saunders SH, Tse ECM, Yates MD, Otero FJ, Trammell SA, Stemp ED, et al. Extracellular DNA promotes efficient extracellular electron transfer by pyocyanin in biofilms *Pseudomonas aeruginosa*. Cell Press. 2020;**182**:919-932. DOI: 10.1016/j.cell.2020.07.006

[13] Saxena P, Joshi Y, Rawat K, Bisht R. Biofilms: Architecture, resistance, quorum sensing and control mechanisms. Indian Journal of Microbiology. 2019;**59**:3-12. DOI: 10.1007/s12088-018-0757-6

[14] Rivera ES, Weiss A, Migas LG, Freiberg JA, Djambazova KV, Neumann EK, et al. Imaging mass spectrometry reveals complex lipid distributions across *Staphylococcus aureus* biofilm layers. Journal of Mass Spectrometry and Advances in the Clinical Lab. 2022;**26**:36-46. DOI: 10.1016/j.jmsacl.2022.09.003

[15] Periasamy S, Joo HS, Duong AC, Bach THL, Tan VY, Chatterjee SS, et al. How *Staphylococcus aureus* biofilms develop their characteristic structure. National Academy of Sciences of the United States of America. 2012;**109**:1281-1286. DOI: 10.1073/pnas.1115006109

[16] Peng Q, Tang X, Dong W, Sun N, Yuan W. A review of biofilm formation of *Staphylococcus aureus* and its regulation mechanism. Antibiotics. 2023;**12**:12. DOI: 10.3390/antibiotics12010012

[17] Fazeli-Nasab B, Sayyed RZ, Mojahed LS, Rahmani AF, Ghafari M, Antonius S. Biofilm production: A strategic mechanism for survival of microbes under stress conditions. Biocatalysis and Agricultural Biotechnology. 2022;**42**:102337. DOI: 10.1016/j.bcab.2022.102337

[18] Karygianni L, Ren Z, Koo H, Thurnheer T. Biofilm matrixome: Extracellular components in structured microbial communities. Trends in Microbiology. 2020;**28**:668-681. DOI: 10.1016/j.tim.2020.03.016

[19] Sauer K, Stoodley P, Goeres DM, Hall-Stoodley L, Burmølle M, Stewart PS, et al. The biofilm life cycle: Expanding the conceptual model of biofilm formation. Nature Reviews Microbiology. 2022;**20**:608-620. DOI: 10.1038/s41579-022-00767-0

[20] Das S. Genetic regulation, biosynthesis and applications of extracellular polysaccharides of the biofilm matrix of bacteria. Carbohydrate Polymers. 2022;**291**:119536. DOI: 10.1016/j.carbpol.2022.119536

[21] Zhao A, Sun J, Liu Y. Understanding bacterial biofilms: From definition to treatment strategies. Frontiers in Cellular and Infection Microbiology. 2023;**13**:1-23. DOI: 10.3389/fcimb.2023.1137947

[22] Mishra A, Aggarwal A, Khan F. Medical device-associated infections caused by biofilm-forming microbial pathogens and controlling strategies. Antibiotics. 2024;**13**:623. DOI: 10.3390/antibióticos13070623

[23] Tran NN, Morrisette T, Jorgensen SCJ, Orench-Benvenutti JM, Kebriaei R. Current therapies and challenges for the treatment of *Staphylococcus aureus* biofilm-related infections. Pharmacotherapy. 2023;**8**:816-832. DOI: 10.1002/phar.2806

[24] Di Ciccio P, Vergara A, Festino AR, Paludi D, Zanardi E, Ghidini S, et al. Biofilm formation by *Staphylococcus aureus* on food contact surfaces: Relationship with temperature and cell surface hydrophobicity. Food Control. 2015;**50**:930-936. DOI: 10.1016/j.foodcont.2014.10.048

[25] Silva V, Pereira JE, Maltez L, Poeta P, Igrejas G. Influence of environmental factors on biofilm formation of *Staphylococci* isolated from wastewater and surface water. Pathogens. 2022;**11**:1069. DOI: 10.3390/patógenos11101069

[26] Wang Z, Chen J, You Z, Liu X, Zhang J. Advances in mechanisms of biofilm formation and drug resistance of *Staphylococcus aureus*. Chinese Journal of Biotechnology. 2024;**40**:2038-2051. DOI: 10.13345/j.cjb.230803

[27] Graf AC, Leonard A, Schäuble M, Becher D, Pané-Farré J, Riedel K. Virulence factors produced by *Staphylococcus aureus* biofilms have a moonlighting function contributing to biofilm integrity. Molecular & Cellular Proteomics. 2019;**18**:1036-1053. DOI: 10.1074/mcp.RA118.001120

[28] Singh S, Singh SK, Chowdhury I, Singh R. Understanding the mechanism of bacterial biofilms resistance to antimicrobial agents. The Open Microbiology Journal. 2017;**11**:53-62. DOI: 10.2174/1874285801711010053

[29] Raafat D, Otto M, Reppschläger K, Iqbal J, Holtfreter S. Fighting *Staphylococcus aureus* biofilms with monoclonal antibodies. Trends in Microbiology. 2019;**27**:303-322. DOI: 10.1016/j.tim.2018.12.009

[30] Sultan AR, Tavakoll M, Lemmens-den TNA, Croughs PD, Verkaik NJ, Verbon A, et al. Real time monitoring of *Staphylococcus aureus* biofilm sensitivity towards antibiotics with isothermal microcalorimetry. PLoS One. 2022;**17**:1-18. DOI: 10.1371/journal.pone.0260272

[31] Oliveira D, Borges A, Rm R, Negrín ZR, Distinto S, Borges F, et al. 2-(2-Methyl-2-nitrovinyl)furan but not furvina interfere with *Staphylococcus aureus Agr* quorum-sensing system and potentiate the action of fusidic acid against biofilms. International Journal of Molecular Sciences. 2021;**22**:613. DOI: 10.3390/ijms22020613

[32] Dauros-Singorenko P, Wiles S, Swift S. *Staphylococcus aureus* biofilms and their response to a relevant in vivo iron source. Frontiers in Microbiology. 2020;**11**:1-16. DOI: 10.3389/fmicb.2020.509525

[33] Lai CKC, Ng RWY, Leung SSY, Hui M, Ip M. Overcoming the rising incidence and evolving mechanisms of antibiotic resistance by novel drug delivery approaches – An overview. Advanced Drug Delivery Reviews. 2022;**181**:1-19. DOI: 10.1016/j.addr.2021.114078

[34] Liu J, Yang L, Hou Y, Soteyome T, Zeng B, Su J, et al. Transcriptomics study on *Staphylococcus aureus* biofilm under low concentration of ampicillin. Frontiers in Microbiology. 2018;**9**:2413. DOI: 10.3389/fmicb.2018.02413

[35] Wu S, Liu Y, Lei L, Zhang H. Antisense yycG regulation of antibiotic sensitivity of methicillin-resistant *Staphylococcus aureus* in chronic osteomyelitis. Surgical Infections. 2019;**20**:1-8. DOI: 10.1089/sur.2019.016

[36] Wu S, Zhang J, Peng Q, Liu Y, Lei L, Zhang H. The role of *Staphylococcus aureus* YycFG in gene regulation, biofilm organization and drug resistance. Antibiotics. 2021;**10**:1555. DOI: 10.3390/antibiotics10121555

[37] Wood TK. Strategies for combating *persister* cell and biofilm infections. Microbial Biotechnology. 2017;**10**:1054-1056. DOI: 10.1111/1751-7915.12774

[38] Waters EM, Rowe SE, O'gara JP, Conlon BP. Convergence of *Staphylococcus aureus* persister and biofilm research: Can biofilms be defined as communities of adherent persister cells? PLOS Pathogens. 2016;**12**:1-5. DOI: 10.1371/journal.ppat.1006012

[39] Miyaue M, Suzuki E, Komiyama Y, Kondo Y, Morikawa M, Maeda S. Bacterial memory of *persisters*: Bacterial *persister* cells can retain their phenotype for days or weeks after withdrawal from colony-biofilm culture. Frontiers in Microbiology. 2018;**26**:1396. DOI: 10.3389/fmicb.2018.01396

[40] Conlon BP, Rowe SE, Gandt AB, Nuxoll AS, Donegan NP, Zalis EA, et al. Persister formation in *Staphylococcus aureus* is associated with ATP depletion. Nature Microbiology. 2016;**1**:16051. DOI: 10.1038/nmicrobiol.2016.51

[41] Yamada KJ, Kielian T. Biofilm-leukocyte cross-talk: Impact on immune polarization and immunometabolism. Journal of Innate Immunity. 2019;**11**:280-288. DOI: 10.1159/000492680

[42] Scherr TD, Heim CE, Morrison JM, Kielian T. Hiding in plain sight: Interplay between staphylococcal biofilms and host immunity. Frontiers in Microbiology. 2014;**5**:1-7. DOI: 10.3389/fimmu.2014.00037

[43] Wells M, Schneider R, Bhattarai B, Currie H, Chavez B, Christopher G, et al. Perspective: The viscoelastic properties of biofilm infections and mechanical interactions with phagocytic immune cells. Frontiers in Cellular and Infection Microbiology. 2023;**16**:1-10. DOI: 10.3389/fcimb.2023.1102199

[44] Archer NK, Mazaitis MJ, Costerton JW, Leid JG, Powers ME, Shirtliff ME. *Staphylococcus aureus* biofilms: Properties, regulation and roles in human disease. Virulence. 2011;**2**:445-459. DOI: 10.4161/viru.2.5.17724

[45] Li M, Yu J, Guo G, Shen H. Interactions between macrophages and biofilm during *Staphylococcus aureus* - Associated implant infection: Difficulties and solutions. Journal of Innate Immunity. 2023;**15**:499-515. DOI: 10.1159/000530385

[46] Vidakovic L, Mikhaleva S, Jeckel H, Nisnevich V, Strenger K, Neuhaus K, et al. Biofilm formation on human immune cells is a multicellular predation strategy of vibrio cholerae. Cell Press. 2023;**186**:2690-2704. DOI: 10.1016/j.cell.2023.05.008

[47] Gulati M, Thomas JM, Ennis CL, Hernday AD, Rawat M, Nobile CJ. The bacillithiol pathway is required for biofilm formation in *Staphylococcus aureus*. Microbial Pathogenesis. 2024;**191**:1-9. DOI: 10.1016/j.micpath.2024.106657

[48] Pinto RM, Soares FA, Reis S, Nunes C, Van DP. Innovative strategies toward the disassembly of the EPS matrix in bacterial biofilms. Frontiers in Microbiology. 2020;**11**:1-20. DOI: 10.3389/fmicb.2020.00952

[49] Srinivasan R, Santhakumari S, Poonguzhali P, Geetha M, Dyavaiah M, Xiangmin L. Bacterial biofilm inhibition: A focused review on recent therapeutic strategies for combating the biofilm mediated infections. Frontiers in Microbiology. 2021;**12**:1-19. DOI: 10.3389/fmicb.2021.676458

[50] Xiu W, Shan J, Yang K, Xiao H, Yumen L, Wang L. Recent development of nanomedicine for the treatment of bacterial biofilm infections. Viewpoints. 2020;**2**:1-23. DOI: 10.1002/VIW.20200065

[51] Correia JPP. Avaliação da capacidade de formação de biofilme e resistência à meticilina de isolados de *Staphylococcus* de origem alimentar [Dissertation]. Lisboa: Universidade de Lisboa; 2023

[52] Rodrigues JCP. Sistemas para veiculação localizada de antibióticos na abordagem terapêutica de infecções no osso [Dissertation]. Lisboa: Universidade de Lisboa; 2020

[53] Silvado AS. Biofilme misto em cateter venoso central com ênfase em *Staphylococcus aureus* e *Candida albicans* [Final course work]. Belo Horizonte:

Universidade Federal de Minas Gerais; 2020

[54] Silva MRA. Potencial de formação de biofilme em amostras de isolados clínicos de *Staphylococcus aureus* [Final course work]. João Pessoa: Universidade Federal da Paraíba; 2023

[55] Vestby LK, Gronseth T, Simm R, Nesse LL. Bacterial biofilm and its role in the pathogenesis of disease. Antibiotics. 2020;**9**:59. DOI: 10.3390/antibiotics9020059

[56] Sued-Karam BR, Olivella JGB, Cabral-Oliveira GG, Pereira-Ribeiro PMA. Resistance and virulence factors of the *Staphylococcus aureus* - A brief review. Seven Editora. 2024. DOI: 10.56238/sevened2024.013-005. Available from: https://sevenpublicacoes.com.br/editora/article/view/4774 [Accessed: August 10, 2024]

[57] Kaushik A, Kest H, Sood M, Steussy BW, Thieman C, Gupta S. Biofilm producing methicillin resistant *Staphylococcus aureus* (MRSA) infections in humans: Clinical implications and management. Pathogens. 2024;**13**:1-28. DOI: 10.3390/pathogens13010076

[58] Lara AL. Avaliação da atividade antimicrobiana, antibiofilme e citotoxicidade do óleo essencial de *Cymbopogon martinii* frente a *Staphylococcus aureus*. [Dissertation]. Santa Maria: Universidade Federal de Santa Maria; 2023

[59] Nascimento ECP, Santos PC, Castro SHM. A Incidência da *Staphylococcus aureus* em hospitais: revisão de obra. Brazilian Journal of Implantology and Health Sciences. 2024;**6**:1646-1660. DOI:. DOI: 10.36557/2674-8169.2024v6n5p1646-1660

[60] Jabir DM. Evaluation of the ability of some bacterial species isolated from UTI to form biofilm. Al-Qadisiyah Journal of Pure Science. 2022;**27**:1-14. DOI: 10.29350/qjps.2022.27.1.1492

[61] Xu K, Wang Y, Jian Y, Chen T, Liu Q, Wang H, et al. *Staphylococcus aureus* ST1 promotes persistent urinary tract infection by highly expressing the urease. Frontiers in Microbiology. 2023;**22**:1-15. DOI: 10.3389/fmicb.2023.1101754

[62] Chen K, Peng C, Chi F, Yu C, Yang Q, Li Z. Antibacterial and antibiofilm activities of chlorogenic acid against yersinia enterocolitica. Frontiers in Microbiology. 2022;**13**:1-14. DOI: 10.3389/fmicb.2022.885092

[63] Wu X, Wang H, Xiong J, Yang G-X, Hu J-F, Zhu Q, et al. *Staphylococcus aureus* biofilm: Formulation, regulatory, and emerging natural products-derived therapeutics. Biofilms. 2024;**7**:1-13. DOI: 10.1016/j.bioflm.2023.100175

[64] Ellis JR, Rowley PA. An apparent lack of synergy between degradative enzymes against *Staphylococcus aureus* biofilms. BioRxiv. 2023;**5**:1-19. DOI: 10.1101/2023.10.05.561034

[65] Redman WK, Welch GS, Rumbaugh KP. Differential efficacy of glycoside hydrolases to disperse biofilms. Frontiers in Cellular and Infection Microbiology. 2020;**10**:1-7. DOI: 10.3389/fcimb.2020.00379

[66] Ellis JR, Rowley PA. An apparent lack of synergy between degradative enzymes against *Staphylococcus aureus* biofilms. MicroPublication Biology. 2024;**5**:1-7. DOI: 10.17912/micropub.biology.001119

[67] Lin Q, Sheng M, Tian Y, Li B, Kang Z, Yang Y, et al. Antibiofilm activity and synergistic effects of DNase I and Lysostaphin against *Staphylococcus*

aureus biofilms. Food Quality and Safety. 2024;**8**:1-12. DOI: 10.1093/fqsafe/fyae024

[68] Azeredo J, García P, Drulis-Kawa Z. Targeting biofilms using phages and their enzymes. Current Opinion in Biotechnology. 2021;**68**:251-261. DOI: 10.1016/j.copbio.2021.02.002

[69] Rodrigues LO, Oliveira MS, Polo AB, Gomes TV, Clemente VB, Tavares LCD, et al. Eficiência das nanopartículas poliméricas no controle de bactérias resistentes aos antimicrobianos: uma revisão. In: Morais MJD, Leitão FNC, Deus MBB, Oliveira FS, Araripe MC, editors. Estudos e escrita científica multidisciplinar em ciências da saúde (eBook). 1st ed. Guarujá: Científica Digital; 2024. pp. 73-90. DOI: 10.37885/240115529

[70] Melo RLF, Souza ICC, Carvalho AJR, Bezerra EM, Costa RF. As nanopartículas como ferramentas biológicas: uma revisão exploratória. Research, Society and Development. 2020;**9**:1-18. DOI: 10.33448/rsd-v9i7.4155

[71] Acosta AC, Santos AS, Silva FAG, Medeiros ES, Oliveira HP, Costa MM, et al. Atividade antibacteriana de nanopartículas de polipirrol diante de *Staphylococcus aureus* isolados de amostras de leite de vacas e cabras com mastite. Arquivo Brasileiro de Medicina Veterinária E Zootecnia. 2020;**72**:1047-1050. DOI: 10.1590/1678-4162-10384

[72] Patel A. Metal nanoparticles produced by plants with antibacterial properties against *Staphylococcus aureus*. Brazilian Journal of Biology. 2022;**82**:1-17. DOI: 10.1590/1519-6984.268052

[73] Chung PY, Khoo REY, Liew HS, Low ML. Antimicrobial and antibiofilm activities of Cu(II) Schiff base complexes against methicillin-susceptible and resistant *Staphylococcus aureus*. Annals of Clinical Microbiology and Antimicrobials. 2021;**20**:1-11. DOI: 10.1186/s12941-021-00473-4

[74] da Silva ACF, Roque SM, Duarte MCT, Nakazato G, Durán N, Cogo-Müller K. Modulação da formação de biofilme de *Staphylococcus aureus* por meio de concentrações subinibitórias de nanopartículas de prata biogênicas e sinvastatina. Farmacologia do Futuro. 2024;**4**:3-16. DOI: 10.3390/futurepharmacol4010002

[75] Rosato A, Maggi F, Cianfaglione K, Conti F, Ciaschetti G, Rakotosaona R, et al. Composição química e atividade antibacteriana de sete óleos essenciais incomuns. Journal of Essential Oil Research. 2018;**30**:233-243. DOI: 10.1080/10412905.2018.1442753

[76] Rosato A, Sblano S, Salvagno L, Carocci A, Clodoveo ML, Corbo F, et al. Anti-biofilm inhibitory synergistic effects of combinations of essential oils and antibiotics. Antibiotics. 2020;**9**:1-13. DOI: 10.3390/antibiotics9100637

[77] Balaure PC, Grumezescu AM. Recent advances in surface nanoengineering for biofilm prevention and control. Part II: Active, combined active and passive, and smart bacteria-responsive antibiofilm nanocoatings. Nanomaterials. 2020;**10**:1-30. DOI: 10.3390/nano10081527

[78] Vladkova TG, Staneva AD, Gospodinova DN. Surface engineered biomaterials and ureteral stents inhibiting biofilm formation and encrustation. Surface and Coatings Technology. 2020;**404**:126424. DOI: 10.1016/j.surfcoat.2020.126424

[79] Li W, Thian ES, Wang M, Wang Z, Ren L. Surface design for antibacterial materials: From fundamentals to advanced strategies. Advanced

Science. 2021;**8**:1-23. DOI: 10.1002/advs.202100368

[80] Kumar S, Roy DN, Dey V. A comprehensive review on techniques to create the anti-microbial surface of biomaterials to intervene in biofouling. Colloid Interface Science Communications. 2021;**43**:100464. DOI: 10.1016/j.colcom.2021.100464

[81] Heinonen T, Hargraves S, Georgieva M, Widmann C, Jacquier N. The antimicrobial peptide TAT-RasGAP317-326 inhibits the formation and expansion of bacterial biofilms *in vitro*. Journal of Global Antimicrobial Resistance. 2021;**25**:227-231. DOI: 10.1016/j.jgar.2021.03.022

[82] Nicolas M, Beito B, Oliveira M, Tudela Martins M, Gallas B, Salmain M, et al. Strategies for antimicrobial peptides immobilization on surfaces to prevent biofilm growth on biomedical devices. Antibiotics. 2022;**11**:1-31. DOI: 10.3390/antibiotics11010013

[83] Mitwalli H, Alsahafi R, Balhaddad AA, Weir MD, Xu HHK, Melo MAS. Emerging contact-killing antibacterial strategies for developing anti-biofilm dental polymeric restorative materials. Bioengineering. 2020;**7**:1-25. DOI: 10.3390/bioengineering7030083

[84] Uneputty A, Dávila-Lezama A, Garibo D, Oknianska A, Bogdanchikova N, Hernández-Sánchez JF, et al. Strategies applied to modify structured and smooth surfaces: A step closer to reduce bacterial adhesion and biofilm formation. Colloid Interface Science Communications. 2022;**46**:1-17. DOI: 10.1016/j.colcom.2021.100560

[85] Chang CT, Chen YT, Hsieh YK, Girsang SP, Wang RS, Chang YC, et al. Dual-functional antibiofilm polymer composite for biodegradable medical devices. Materials Science and Engineering: C. 2021;**123**:1-11. DOI: 10.1016/j.msec.2021.111985

[86] Krukiewicz K, Kazek-Kęsik A, Brzychczy-Wloch M, Los MJ, Ateba CN, Mehrbod P, et al. Recent advances in the control of clinically important biofilms. International Journal of Molecular Sciences. 2022;**23**:1-26. DOI: 10.3390/ijms23179526

[87] Jiang R, Hao L, Song L, Tian L, Fan Y, Zhao J, et al. Lotus-leaf-inspired hierarchical structured surface with non-fouling and mechanical bactericidal performances. Chemical Engineering Journal. 2020;**398**:1-12. DOI: 10.1016/j.cej.2020.125609

[88] Wang Y, Yang Y, Shi Y, Song H, Yu C. Antibiotic-free antibacterial strategies enabled by nanomaterials: Progress and perspectives. Advanced Materials. 2020;**32**:1-21. DOI: 10.1002/adma.201904106

[89] Watson GS, Green DW, Schwarzkopf L, Li X, Cribb BW, Myhra S, et al. A gecko skin micro/nano structure – A low adhesion, superhydrophobic, anti-wetting, self-cleaning, biocompatible, antibacterial surface. Acta Biomaterialia. 2015;**21**:109-122. DOI: 10.1016/j.actbio.2015.03.007

[90] Arisoy FD, Kolewe KW, Homyak B, Kurtz IS, Schiffman JD, Watkins JJ. Bioinspired photocatalytic shark-skin surfaces with antibacterial and antifouling activity via nanoimprint lithography. ACS Applied Materials Interfaces. 2018;**10**:20055-20063. DOI: 10.1021/acsami.8b05066

[91] Rigo S, Cai C, Gunkel-Grabole G, Maurizi L, Zhang X, Xu J, et al. Nanoscience-based strategies to engineer antimicrobial surfaces. Advanced

Science. 2018;**5**:1-13. DOI: 10.1002/advs.201700892

[92] Yang X, Zhang W, Qin X, Cui M, Guo Y, Wang T, et al. Recent progress on bioinspired antibacterial surfaces for biomedical application. Biomimetics. 2022;**7**:1-25. DOI: 10.3390/biomimetics7030088

[93] Kranjec C, Angeles MD, Marli TM, Fernández L, García P, Kjos M, et al. Staphylococcal biofilms: Challenges and novel therapeutic perspectives. Antibiotics. 2021;**10**:1-28. DOI: 10.3390/antibiotics10020131

[94] Teixeira CGS, Sanitá PV, Ribeiro APD, Dias LM, Jorge JH, Pavarina AC. Antimicrobial photodynamic therapy effectiveness against susceptible and methicillin-resistant *Staphylococcus aureus* biofilms. Photodiagnosis and Photodynamic Therapy. 2020;**30**:1-9. DOI: 10.1016/j.pdpdt.2020.101760

[95] Parlet CP, Kavanaugh JS, Crosby HA, Raja HA, El-Elimat T, Todd DA, et al. Apicidin attenuates MRSA virulence through quorum-sensing inhibition and enhanced host defense. Cell Reports. 2019;**27**:187-198. DOI: 10.1016/j.celrep.2019.03.018

[96] Swolana D, Kępa M, Kabała-Dzik A, Dzik R, Wojtyczka RD. Sensitivity of *Staphylococcal* biofilm to selected compounds of plant origin. Antibiotics. 2021;**10**:1-13. DOI: 10.3390/antibiotics10050607

[97] Scaldaferri L, Tameirão ER, Flores SA, Neves RASC, Correia TS, Carmo JR, et al. Formas de resistência microbiana e estratégias para minimizar sua ocorrência na terapia antimicrobiana. Pubvet Medicina Veterináris e Zootecnia. 2020;**14**:1-10. DOI: 10.31533/pubvet.v14n8a621.1-10

[98] Josephs-Spaulding J, Singh OV. Medical device sterilization and reprocessing in the era of multidrug-resistant (MDR) bacteria: Issues and regulatory concepts. Frontiers in Medical Technology. 2021;**2**:1-15. DOI: 10.3389/fmedt.2020.587352

[99] Ayub A, Cheong YK, Castro JC, Cumberlege O, Chrysanthou A. Use of hydrogen peroxide vapour for microbiological disinfection in hospital environments: A review. Bioengineering. 2024;**11**:1-16. DOI: 10.3390/bioengineering11030205

[100] Su Y, Yrastorza JT, Matis M, Cusick J, Zhao S, Wang G, et al. Biofilms: Formation, research models, potential targets, and methods for prevention and treatment. Advanced Science. 2022;**9**:1-36. DOI: 10.1002/advs.202203291

[101] Ciarolla AA, Lapin N, Williams D, Chopra R, Greenberg DE. Physical approaches to prevent and treat bacterial biofilm. Antibiotics. 2022;**12**:1-24. DOI: 10.3390/antibiotics12010054

[102] Maillard JY, Centeleghe I. How biofilm changes our understanding of cleaning and disinfection. Antimicrobial Resistance & Infection Control. 2023;**12**:1-11. DOI: 10.1186/s13756-023-01290-4

Chapter 3

Recent Trends and Advances in Design of Rapid Tests for Colorimetric Detection of *Staphylococcus aureus*

Cemile Yilmaz, Cagla Celik, Nilay Ildiz, Esma Eryilmaz-Eren, Mehmet Akif Dündar, Uner Kayabas and Ismail Ocsoy

Abstract

Staphylococcus aureus (*S. aureus*), which is a member of Micrococcacease family, is one of the most dangerous disease-causing bacteria. *S. aureus* is also the biggest factor causing hospital-acquired infections worldwide, as well as life-threatening infections such as meningitis, septicaemia, and suppurating wounds in the human body. Today, there have been various phenotypic and/or genotypic methods for the detection of both *S. aureus* and methicillin-resistant *S. aureus* (MRSA) strains. Although genotypic methods have been commonly used for certain and rapid results, they are quite expensive and rarely available in all hospitals; they need costly and complicated devices and expert use. To address these issues, researchers have recently developed nanomaterials (NMs) and organic molecules-based phenotypic methods for rapid, sensitive, and economical detection of *S. aureus* and MRSA. We focus on evaluating colorimetric assays using NMs and pH indicator-containing tests for the rapid, sensitive, and cost-effective detection of *S. aureus* and MRSA, and specifically target their application in both clinical and environmental contexts.

Keywords: rapid test, phenotypic testing, colorimetic response, antibiotic resistant bacteria, *Staphylococcus aureus*

1. Introduction

Staphylococcus aureus is a leading pathogen responsible for both community and hospital-associated bacteraemia. It is a facultative anaerobic Gram-positive coccus commonly found as a commensal organism in the respiratory tract and on the skin [1, 2]. Despite its typical role as a harmless colonizer, *S. aureus* can cause infections ranging from mild skin infections to severe, life-threatening diseases such as bacteraemia. Bacteraemia caused by *S. aureus* is particularly serious and is associated with high morbidity and mortality, even with appropriate treatment [3]. In paediatric patients, especially those in intensive care units, *S. aureus* is a significant cause of several infections. Common infections in children include sepsis, toxic shock syndrome, osteomyelitis, septic arthritis, pneumonia, and skin and soft tissue infections. Neonates in intensive care units are particularly vulnerable, with bloodstream infections often associated with umbilical or central venous catheters. Staphylococcal scalded skin syndrome, characterized by generalized erythematous blistering, is particularly severe in neonates due to the lack of protective exotoxin antibodies [4, 5].

The clinical importance of *S. aureus* is underscored by its role in both community and healthcare settings and the growing challenge of antimicrobial resistance. Methicillin-resistant *S. aureus* (MRSA) outbreaks in neonatal intensive care units highlight the continued need for robust infection control measures [6]. Epidemiologic data from The Centers for Disease Control and Prevention's 2023 report indicate that African Americans have higher rates of invasive MRSA infection than Caucasians. The increasing incidence of MRSA in both hospital and community settings underscores the critical need for continued vigilance in infection prevention and management strategies [7].

2. Detection of *Staphylococcus aureus*

Rapid and accurate detection of bacterial presence, concentration, and identity (type) in the environment, as well as food and clinical samples, is vital for both public health security and early diagnosis of infectious infections [8, 9]. In this sense, there are various classical techniques for the detection and identification of bacterial pathogens. For example, culture and colony counting, immunological approaches, polymerase chain reaction (PCR) and reverse transcriptase polymerase chain reaction (RT-PCR), flow cytometry, mass spectrometry, microarrays, fluorescence-based assay, and electrochemical-based assay have been developed and are still in use. However, although these techniques provide accurate and sensitive results, the most important disadvantages of these techniques are that they are time-consuming, complicated, and laborious, require complicated tools, and are not suitable for field work (portability) [10–22].

A variety of tools including targeting ligand conjugated NPs, enzyme incorporated systems, and paper-based assays, have been developed for colorimetric detection, profiling, and destruction of *S. aureus* and MRSA. In response to these challenges, recent advancements have focused on developing novel methods utilizing nanomaterials (NMs) and pH indicators for the rapid, sensitive, and economical detection of *S. aureus* and MRSA. This work aims to explore the efficacy of colorimetric assays and nanomaterial-based approaches for the detection and profiling of *S. aureus* and MRSA, addressing the need for more accessible, efficient, and portable diagnostic tools. The study seeks to evaluate the performance of these innovative methods in various clinical and environmental contexts, enhancing early detection and improving public health outcomes.

2.1 Nanoparticles-based colorimetric detection of *Staphylococcus aureus*

In recent years, gold nanoparticles (Au NPs) have been frequently used in the fields of electronics and optics, especially in bioanalytical and biomedical fields, thanks to their unique properties. Au NPs have more advantageous properties than others like easy synthesis, short production time, stable structure (can be stored at focal temperature for a long time), high surface area, easy attachment of functional groups to the surface and most importantly, unique optical properties. Au NPs are used quite actively in applications in the field of bionanotechnology due to their excellent optical properties. Au NPs have begun to be used as biosensors due to the plasmon resonances that they create in the visible region when they interact with light. When Au NPs interact with an analyte, the presence of the analyte and its concentration in the environment can be measured by the change in the optical properties of Au NPs [10, 23–29].

S. aureus can cause infections ranging from simple food poisoning to life-threatening invasive infections [30]. It can escape the host immune response and causes these infections by producing biofilms and antiphagocytic capsules, persisting intracellularly, and inhibiting leukocyte chemotaxis. *S. aureus* may cause skin and soft tissue infections (such as impetigo, folliculitis, furuncle, carbuncle, and cellulitis) as well as necrotizing fasciitis by invading muscle and fascia. It infects bones and joints, causing septic arthritis and osteomyelitis. In the literature, *S. aureus* is reported as a causative agent of severe necrotizing pneumonia in immunocompromised or alcoholic patients [31–35]. In addition, MRSA is the main causative agent of hospital-acquired invasive infections. It forms a biofilm that causes bacteraemia associated with infections associated with invasive devices (such as intravenous catheters) and difficult-to-treat infections of artificial heart valve endocarditis [36–38]. MRSA also leads to surgical site infections, one of the most important complications of surgical procedures [39–41]. *S. aureus* also has exotoxins. Food poisoning and toxic shock syndrome are infections caused by staph aureus through its toxins [42].

Penicillinase synthesis is present in more than 95% of staphylococcal strains worldwide; therefore, penicillin is not a treatment option. Penicillinase-resistant penicillins (methicillin, nafcillin, and oxacillin) and quinolones may be used in local infections or if susceptible based on antimicrobial resistance test results [43, 44]. First-generation cephalosporins (such as cefazolin and cephalothin) are also options for surgical prophylaxis, depending on local antimicrobial resistance data. Ceftaroline and ceftabiprole are fifth-generation cephalosporins and are effective against MRSA. Methicillin-resistant bacteria are resistant to all beta-lactams, including cephalosporins [45–47]. Vancomycin is a glycopeptide and should be the first choice in the presence of MRSA bacteraemia or penicillin allergy in MSSA. Teicoplanin is another glycopeptide that penetrates tissues better than vancomycin [48]. Daptomycin is a cyclic lipopeptide antibiotic and is effective against biofilm. Indicated for MRSA bacteraemia if vancomycin-induced nephrotoxicity is present [49, 50]. Dalbavancin and oritavancin are lipoglycopeptide antibiotics newly approved by the FDA for skin and skin structure infections caused by MRSA [51]. Linezolid is a bacteriostatic antibiotic that can be used to treat MRSA bacteraemia, skin infections and pneumonia where other treatments are contraindicated [52]. In biofilm-associated infections such as endocarditis and osteomyelitis, combination therapy with rifampin or aminoglycosides may be considered [53].

S. aureus is a pyogenic bacteria and is seen with many polymorphonuclear leukocytes in the staining of samples taken from the infection site. It grows rapidly on blood agar, forming cream and gold colonies and causing beta haemolysis. Although the gold standard method for diagnosis is culture, it requires a long time. Rapid tests are needed. MALDI-TOF is a common system used routinely to identify *S. aureus* from positive blood cultures. Fluorescent-based tests that detect antigens and anti-*S. aureus* antibodies, tissue rapid PCR detection tests, are rapid tests that are in the development phase. Detection of aureus exotoxins in foods and milk is important for the food industry [54–56].

Recent advancements in nanotechnology are revolutionizing early and precise diagnostics in healthcare. Biosensors based on NMs integrate critical elements such as bioreceptors, transducers, signal processors, and display mechanisms. These sensors benefit from the extensive surface areas and enhanced conductivity of NMs, which enable effective, robust, and reliable biomolecule detection [57]. For instance, the use of Au and silver (Ag) nanomaterials in colorimetric sensors has shown significant improvements in detecting pathogens like MRSA. These NMs amplify colorimetric signals through mechanisms like aggregation, morphological changes, and surface reactions, offering an expanded surface area for biomolecular probe attachment, which enhances signal strength and overall detection accuracy [58]. Various types of sensors, including electrochemical, fluorescent, and mechanical, have been developed to identify MRSA biomarkers, demonstrating effective performance in clinical environments [59].

Colorimetric sensors based on NMs stand out for their ease of use and visual clarity, allowing results to be interpreted without complex instrumentation. NM-based colorimetric sensors combine traditional and innovative techniques, significantly enhancing detection capabilities. The limitations of conventional colorimetric tests, which often suffer from sensitivity and specificity issues, are mitigated by the use of metallic NPs. These NPs provide large surface areas that improve colour change detection and signal clarity by facilitating the binding of recognition molecules like antibodies or enzymes [60].

The application of NMs for pathogen detection is particularly prominent in colorimetric assays. These sensors utilize the electrostatic aggregation properties of NPs to induce detectable colour changes. Au and Ag NPs are particularly effective in this role, enabling straightforward visual detection [61]. Recent reviews highlight the potential of NP-based colorimetric sensors for detecting *S. aureus*, emphasizing their heightened sensitivity and specificity. By leveraging the high surface-to-volume ratio and reactivity of metal NPs, these sensors offer rapid and accurate pathogen detection through observable colorimetric shifts [62]. Plasmonic NPs are central to the development of rapid colorimetric sensors for bacterial pathogen detection. These sensors generally rely on colour changes caused by NP aggregation or anti-aggregation effects. However, external variables can sometimes lead to false positives, affecting the reliability and selectivity of the methods [58]. To improve performance, innovative approaches such as anti-aggregation techniques and chemical etching are used to refine the plasmonic properties of the NPs. These advancements enhance the sensors' ability to detect pathogens like *S. aureus* swiftly, sensitively, and cost-effectively [57].

Yuan et al. [63] developed an Au NP-based colorimetric sensor for detecting *S. aureus* using aptamer recognition and tiramine signal amplification (TSA). Biotinylated aptamers specifically bind *S. aureus* to microtitre plates. Through TSA, a large amount of catalase enzyme binds to the bacteria's surface, accelerating H_2O_2 consumption and turning the solution blue. In the absence of the target bacterium, the solution turns red. The sensor is highly selective for *S. aureus* because the aptamers bind specifically to unique surface markers on *S. aureus*, distinguishing it from other bacteria. This method offers a faster and more sensitive alternative compared to other techniques, with a detection sensitivity of 9 CFU mL^{-1} for *S. aureus*.

Shahbazi et al. [59] developed a new method for detecting *S. aureus* DNA by employing Au NP in a colorimetric assay. This technique offers quick detection, taking only 10–15 minutes (min), with a noticeable colour shift that can be observed both visually and through UV-Vis spectroscopy. The assay's sensitivity surpassed that of the PCR method, detecting DNA at lower concentrations (8.73 ng/µL compared to 30 ng/µL). The method demonstrated a broad linear detection range, high specificity, and precise accuracy in identifying *S. aureus* DNA, with Au NPs having a higher aspect ratio proving particularly advantageous. Additionally, this approach proved effective in quantifying target DNA in food and clinical samples, suggesting its potential for on-site detection of *S. aureus*.

A variety of organic and biological targeting agents have been synthesized to specifically detect bacteria and attached to Au NPs, enabling both visual and spectrometric detection of bacteria. For example, Dr DeGrasse developed specific oligonucleic acids called "aptamers" for the enterotoxin B protein found in *S. aureus*. This specifically selected DNA sequence was intended to selectively bind to enterotoxin B and thus recognize *S. aureus* [56]. Dr Chen and co-workers attempted to colorimetrically detect *S. aureus* by attaching the selected aptamer for enterotoxin B protein to Au NPs [64]. DNA or RNA aptamers have been produced by Cell-Systematic Evolution of Ligands by Exponential Enrichment (Cell-SELEX) technology to select aptamers for *S. aureus* and its methicillin-resistant isolate [65–68]. Recently, ligands containing boronic acid groups have been extensively used to increase the selectivity and sensitivity in bacterial detection. For example, Dr Wang and co-workers used disulphide phenylboronic acid on Au NPs and used this conjugated structure for colorimetric determination of *S. aureus*. Disulphide phenylboronic acids on gold nano-spheres bind covalently to cis-diol groups on glycans, forming the wall of S. aureus and stable complexes. However, the biggest disadvantage of the system is that there is only one boronic acid unit in the disulphide phenylboronic acid used and it also weakens the selectivity, sensitivity and binding strength of the system to bacteria [69].

2.2 Catalytic activity-based colorimetric detection of *Staphylococcus aureus*

S. aureus is a leading cause of both healthcare-associated and community-acquired infections. This bacterium poses a significant health risk due to its virulence factors, including endotoxins, which can lead to severe conditions such as endocarditis, pneumonia, meningitis, toxic shock syndrome, and sepsis. Prompt identification of the infection is crucial for effective treatment. Several diagnostic approaches exist for detecting pathogenic bacteria, including culture methods, biochemical assays, enzyme-linked immunosorbent assays (ELISA), and polymerase chain reaction (PCR) [70].

All of these techniques are limited by their lengthy processing times, low sensitivity, and the need for intricate sample preparation [71]. Consequently, there is an urgent need for a highly sensitive and rapid approach to detect *S. aureus* effectively. Recently, there has been extensive research into biosensors. In contrast to conventional techniques, nanotechnology-based biosensors offer enhanced speed, improved efficiency, and greater accuracy [72].

Peroxidase-mimicking activity has gained significant attention for identifying pathogenic bacteria because it offers benefits like cost-effectiveness, ease of use, quick results, and no need for costly instruments. The appearance of a blue colour, resulting from the catalytic oxidation of 3,3′,5,5′-tetramethylbenzidine (TMB) by H_2O_2 in a paper-based assay, is easily observable with the naked eye. Hence, there is a pressing demand for developing a novel colorimetric technique for the precise and selective identification of pathogenic microorganisms. Colorimetric biosensors, which rely on observable colour changes, are highly effective for detecting a wide range of targets and biomolecules. Their appeal lies in their visible colour shifts, straightforward operation, and rapid results [73].

Peroxidases represent a broad category of enzymes that facilitate the oxidation-reduction reactions dependent on H_2O_2, thereby mitigating the harmful effects of peroxides and certain aromatic compounds (electron donors). Additionally, these enzymes can drive the transformation of chromogenic substrates into coloured products that can be measured using spectrophotometric techniques. Consequently, peroxidases are extensively utilized in biochemical assays [74]. Hosseini [75] introduced a novel, rapid, and highly sensitive colorimetric approach for detecting S. aureus by utilizing DNA-templated nanoclusters as bioreceptors to identify whole bacterial cells for the first time. The method is highly specific to *S. aureus* because the aptamers in the nanoclusters bind only to *S. aureus*, while other bacteria like *Salmonella Typhimurium, Escherichia coli, and Pseudomonas aeruginosa* do not trigger the same response. This technique was successfully employed for the selective detection of bacterial cells in samples of milk, orange juice, and human serum, ensuring accurate detection even in complex samples.

The present study is a straightforward and dependable colorimetric assay for the sensitive and selective detection of *S. aureus*, utilizing IgY-Fe_3O_4/Au nanocomposites as capture probes and apt-AuNPs as optical signal enhancers. The assay leverages the enhanced catalytic properties of Au NPs, achieved through etching, combined with a TMB/H_2O_2 reporting system. This approach significantly improves the catalytic performance of the modified Au NPs, leading to a greater signal difference between positive and negative samples. The IgY antibodies and thiol-modified aptamers are specifically designed to target and bind to unique surface proteins of *S. aureus*. This selective binding inhibits the catalytic activity of the modified Au NPs, ensuring that only the presence of *S. aureus* leads to the observed colorimetric response, allowing for precise detection even in complex matrices. *S. aureus* detection is possible with a low limit of detection (LOD) of 10 CFU/mL and a broad linear range extending from 10 to 10^6 CFU/mL. Yao et al. [76] developed a colorimetric immunoassay for rapid *S. aureus* detection that incorporates etching-enhanced peroxidase-like activity of Au NPs, utilizing IgY-Fe_3O_4/Au nanocomposites and apt-AuNPs to amplify optical signals. This method facilitates easy visual detection of *S. aureus* at a minimal LOD of 10 CFU/mL and covers a wide detection range from 10 to 10^6 CFU/mL as shown in **Figure 1**.

Zhang et al. [77] developed a single-step colorimetric assay for detecting S. aureus by utilizing the peroxidase-like activity of Apt-Fe_3O_4/Au nanocomposites (NCs), achieving high specificity through the aptamer's selective binding to a unique *S. aureus* surface target, with a low detection limit of 10 CFU/mL and a broad linear range from 10 to 10^6 CFU/mL in just 12 minutes. Gao et al. [78] successfully developed porous nanozymes with an Au core and platinum (Pt) shell (Au@PtNEs) that exhibit high peroxidase-like activity and robustness. They employed a double-recognition colorimetric assay that does not require washing for the rapid and specific detection of *S. aureus*. This approach achieved a detection limit of 40 CFU/mL and covered a range from 5×10^{-1} to 5×10^{-5} CFU/mL within 1.5 hours.

Liu et al. [79] engineered a new multimetal hybrid Fe_3O_4-Ag-MnO_2 NC, using trisodium citrate for stabilization. They successfully created spherical Fe_3O_4 NPs that are stable, water-soluble, and decorated with carboxyl groups. The resulting colorimetric technique proved highly effective for detecting *S. aureus* in various food matrices. Additionally, they developed a smartphone-based colorimetric platform employing an enzyme cascade amplification strategy to identify *S. aureus* in milk. This system involved a cascade bio-nanozyme setup with glucose oxidase (GOx) immobilized on Fe_3O_4@Ag. The method utilized a cascade reaction initiated by H_2O_2, generated through glucose oxidation by GOx, and subsequent colour generation through the natural peroxidase-like activity of Fe_3O_4@Ag with TMB. *S. aureus* detection was feasible through visual inspection and smartphone measurement, with the platform achieving a low detection limit of 6.9 CFU/mL in just 50 min and demonstrating commendable specificity and sensitivity.

Duan et al. [80] introduced an innovative nanozyme, PHCS@CuNcPOPTP, which exhibits light-responsive oxidase-like activity through a unique chain-linking approach. This organic-inorganic hybrid nanocomposite was synthesized using a

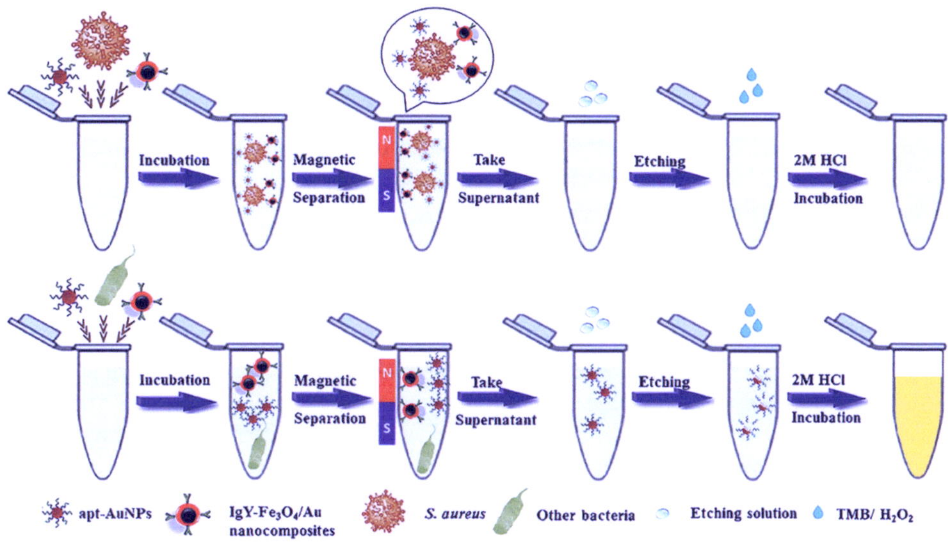

Figure 1.
Schematic of a colorimetric assay for detecting S. aureus *using etching-enhanced gold nanoparticles with IgY-Fe_3O_4/Au nanocomposites and apt-AuNPs for improved signal differentiation [76].*

single-step Friedel-Crafts alkylation reaction. The resulting material demonstrated exceptional light-driven catalytic properties due to its distinctive sensitivity to light. PHCS@CuNcPOPTP served as a base for constructing various signal probes, such as PHCS@CuNcPOPTP@Au-Ab2/DNA1, PHCS@CuNcPOPTP@Au-DNA1, and PHCS@CuNcPOPTP@Au-DNA2, which incorporated rabbit anti-*S. aureus* Rosenbach tropina antibody (bs-4582R, Ab2), DNA1, and DNA2, respectively. By repeatedly hybridizing DNA with these probes, a large quantity of PHCS@ CuNcPOPTP-DNA dendrimers was generated, facilitating a chromogenic reaction without needing high H_2O_2 concentrations. This approach led to significant catalytic enhancement and minimized background interference. The resulting detection system demonstrated high sensitivity with a broad linear range (from 10^1 to 10^8 CFU/mL) and an impressive limit of detection (LOD) of 3.40 CFU/mL.

2.3 Paper-based colorimetric detection of *Staphylococcus aureus*

Paper is often the preferred substrate in biosensor design. It has many advantages [81–83]. Paper is easy to access and cost-effective. These properties make it suitable for large-scale production. Due to its lightweight nature, it can be easily transported and stored. The cellulosic structure of paper allows molecules to be carried by capillary action. This permits aptamers, antibodies, and various biomolecules to migrate easily. Therefore, paper as a substrate can be easily modified into a sensor. In addition, paper-based sensors can be easily disposed of without the risk of biohazard contamination from incineration.

Microfluidic devices were first developed in 1979 [84]. They allow measurements to be taken from the sample on a micrometer scale. Multiple functions such as sample introduction, mixing, reaction and signal output can operate in one single unit. The advantages include miniaturization, a smaller sample volume requirement, a lower consumption of materials and a lower cost. It also allows point-of-care (POC)/point-of-use (POU) diagnostics with lab-on-a-chip technology. The development of microfluidic devices has been in the direction of paper-based microfluidics for improved sensitivity, selectivity, and portability. In particular, paper-based microfluidic analytical devices (μPAD) have played an important role in the development of biosensor devices in low-resource settings (e.g. LMICs) since it was first proposed by the Whitesides group in 2007 [85].

As a result of developments, μPADs generate a signal output using a variety of sensing methods such as magnetic, optical, distance, and temperature-based readout. These sensing capabilities allow them to detect microorganisms as whole cells. In addition, pathogen nucleic acids and other biomarkers such as antigens, metabolites and toxins can also be detected using these techniques. Following the publication by the Whitesides group [86], it is now possible to sensitively detect pathogens in a wide range of samples.

Over the past decades, since μPAD was first reported by the Whitesides group in 2007 [85], studies have shown that its potential for mass production and commercialization is very promising. In addition to being cost-effective, accessible and stable, its porous structure allows for easy modification with various chemical and biological reagents. The capillary effect allows the movement of molecules without the need for an external power supply. The white background color allows excellent colorimetric detection and makes the difference visible to the eye [81–83].

μPAD can provide colourimetric, fluorescent and chemiluminescent signals by optical [86–90] and electrochemical [91, 92] methods. Sensitivity and selectivity have been enhanced by the use of technologies such as nanotechnology and the CRISPR/Cas system. Thus, there has been an expansion in the areas of application for μPAD. Suea-Ngam et al. [90] developed a colorimetric test for the detection of MRSA that provides rapid, sensitive and quantitative results. The colorimetric test was developed as a silver nanoplate (Ag NPls)-based μPAD. The researchers were able to obtain a qualitative colourimetric result with the naked eye. They were also able to perform a quantitative analysis using a smartphone camera. The test gives results in 30 min and a linear response (R2 = 0.994) was obtained between 1 and 104 copies.

A new generation of NM-based detection methods has been developed with the advance of technologies such as microfluidics and NMs. Paper-based sensors prepared in the form of lateral flow assays (LFA) provide colorimetric results with NMs. In particular, Au NPs and silver nanoparticles (Ag NP) are used. The localized surface plasmon resonance (LSPR) properties of the mentioned metallic NPs are utilized. For example, Lu et al. developed an aptamer-based LFA test for the detection of *S. Typhimurium, E. coli O157:H7, and S. aureus*. The color change is based on AuNPs. The ability of AuNPs to appear red in colloidal form and purple in aggregated form has been utilized. Colorimetric response can be observed by eye after 10 min incubation [93, 94].

Guo et al. [95] developed a test for the detection of pathogens in infected wounds that can perform rapid sampling, photocontrolled release and SERS detection. The triple-function adhesive tape can detect *P. aeruginosa* and *S. aureus*. It can detect bacteria directly from the wound after several hours of incubation. This test shows great promise for use as a POC test device.

Wang et al. [96] studied the simultaneous detection of *Acinetobacter baumannii* (AB), *E.coli* (EC) and multidrug-resistant *S. aureus* (SA). The developed test provides results in 35 min and is a μPAD containing dual aptamers. In the developed test, aptamers were first fixed to the paper layer of the sensor by UV crosslinking and blocking. Secondly, an aptamer-biotin conjugate was conjugated. Finally, HRP-streptavidin and TMB were applied. A blue color change was observed in the presence of bacteria. The LOD was visible to the naked eye even at 10-fold serial dilutions.

Nanoclusters have been used for the detection of *S. aureus* due to their nanozyme activity. Bagheri Pebdeni et al. synthesized Au/Pt bimetallic nanoclusters using cytosine-rich single-stranded DNA for the detection of *S. aureus*. Au/Pt bimetallic nanoclusters oxidized TMB in the presence of H_2O_2 due to their peroxidation properties. When TMB is oxidized, specific areas of the sensor change color from clear to dark blue. The catalytic activity of the nanoclusters is reduced in the presence of bacteria. This leads to the production of less oxidized TMB, and consequently, the intensity of the blue color decreases [75]. The working mechanism of this paper-based sensor is shown in **Figure 2**.

Suaifan et al. developed an assay based on the proteolytic activity of *S. aureus*. The assay detects proteolytic activity using a magnetic nanobond peptide probe immobilized on a gold platform [97].

A paper-based sensor array capable of detecting sepsis in children was developed by Sheini et al. The working mechanism of the sensor array is based on measuring changes in the optical or electrical properties of the indicator after interaction with bacteria or metabolites released during bacterial growth. Au and Ag metal nanoclusters were immobilized on Whatman paper. The developed sensor was used to detect pathogens in pediatric serum samples. It detects sepsis-causing bacteria such as *S. aureus, Streptococcus pyogenes, E. coli*, and *P. aeruginosa.* Changes in fluorescence emission intensity in the presence of the pathogen were recorded in less than 15 seconds using a UV lamp and a smartphone. The researchers quantitatively analyzed the color changes using ImageJ software. The detection limit was 80 CFU/mL and a linear calibration curve was obtained in the range 10^2–10^8 CFU/mL. This test enables the diagnosis of bacteria in human serum and the detection of *S. aureus* in food samples such as milk, orange juice, and human serum [98]. The colorimetric changes of this sensor array in the presence of bacteria are shown in **Figure 3**.

In a study by Sekar et al. in 2024, 6 different pathogens were detected using glucose-functionalized gold nanoparticles. Phyto-synthesized AuNPs (Glu-AuNPs) act as transducers. The color intensity of the paper-based colorimetric sensor increased with bacterial concentration and was measured with Adobe Photoshop software. This sensor is suitable for measurement of real samples [99].

Another study in the same year developed a novel paper biosensor based on a polydiacetylene (PDA) polymer functionalized with fibrinogen (**Figure 4**) [100]. The fluorophore property is released by proteins that bind to fibrinogen on the surface of *S. aureus.* The binding causes the PDA to bend, resulting in changes in color and fluorescence. The detection limit was 50.1 CFU/mL for *S. aureus*-contaminated food samples and 65.0 CFU/mL for the pure *S. aureus* culture. Mechanism of the working principle is shown in **Figure 4**.

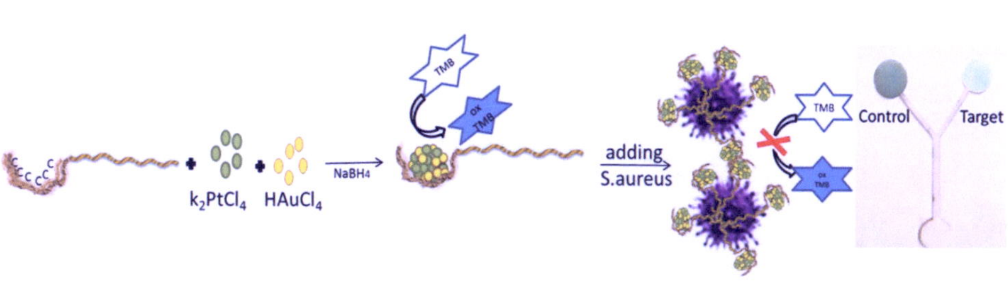

Figure 2.
Schematic of a paper-based sensor with Au/Pt bimetallic nanoclusters for detecting S. aureus, *demonstrating reduced colour intensity due to decreased catalytic activity in the presence of bacteria [75].*

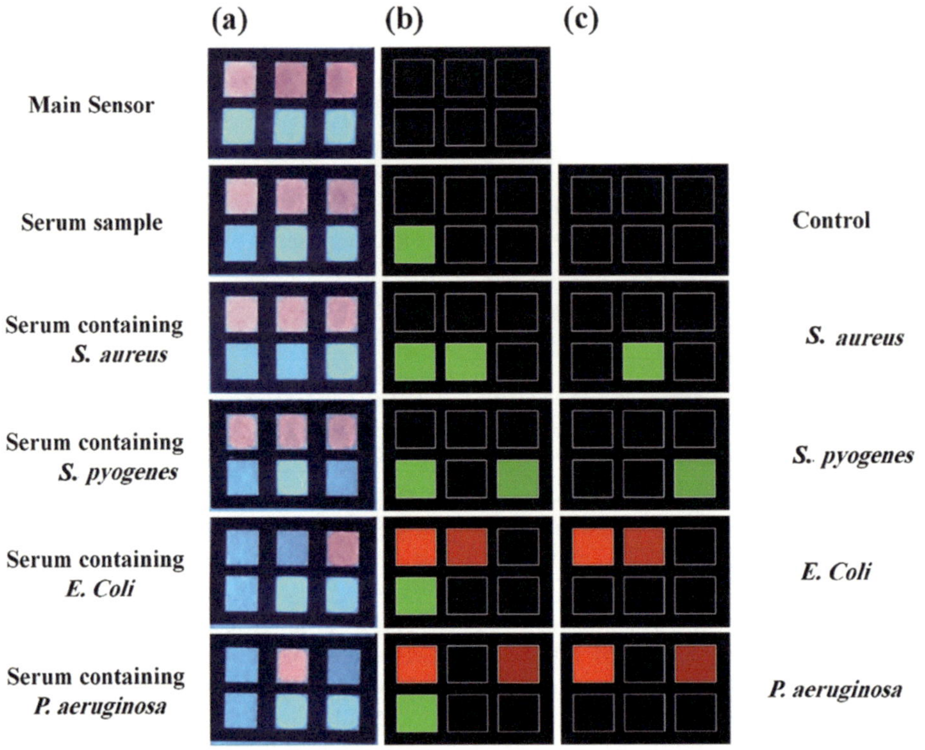

Figure 3.
A fluorimetric, paper-based sensor array for the detection of paediatric sepsis, utilizing Au and Ag nanoclusters to detect sepsis-causing bacteria such as S. aureus, S. pyogenes, E. Coli *and* P. aeruginosa *in serum samples. The figure shows (a) the layout of the sensor array, (b) the fluorescence emission changes recorded upon exposure to bacteria, and (c) the quantitative analysis of colour changes using ImageJ software [98].*

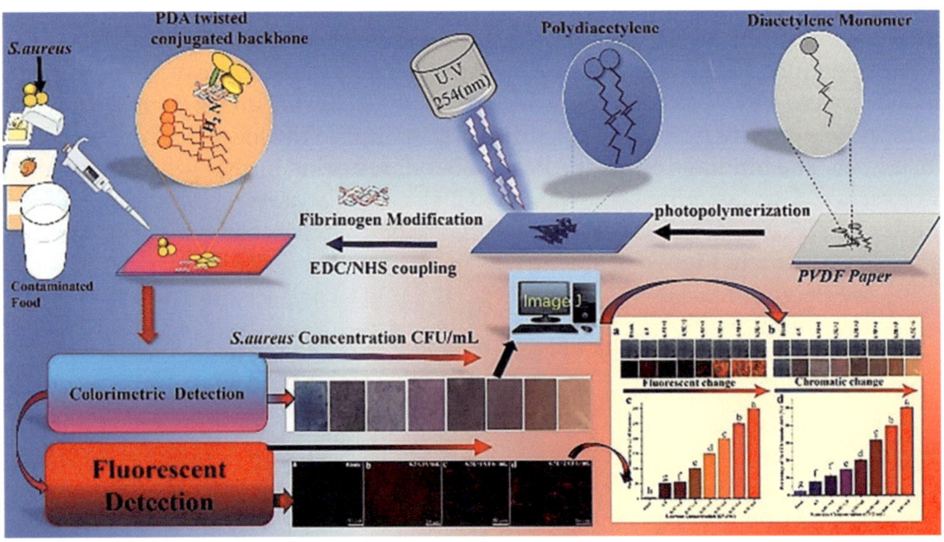

Figure 4.
Fabrication steps and working mechanism of a paper-based biosensor for S. aureus *detection, utilizing a polydiacetylene (PDA) polymer functionalized with fibrinogen, resulting in colour and fluorescence changes upon bacterial binding [100].*

In one of the recent studies, direct loop-mediated isothermal amplification (LAMP) and LFA were combined to detect *S. aureus*. The limit of detection was 10^2 CFU/ml with no cross-reactivity with other strains. POC technologies can become more widespread thanks to this developed system. It has advantages such as short test time, high sensitivity and user-friendly application [101].

3. Conclusion

Pathogenic (disease-causing) bacteria, especially those in the gram-positive group, very easily live and multiply in the environment and cause serious diseases. Studies have shown that *S. aureus* colonizes in nose and throat mucosa of ~30% and ~ 20% of healthy people, respectively. *S. aureus* has created isolates resistant to antibiotics, resulting in infections that are very difficult to treat and can lead to death. Detection and elimination of these bacteria are important not only for human and animal health, but also for industrial and plant production safety. Therefore, this review focuses on recent studies on the development of new diagnostic tests for the detection of *S. aureus* and MRSA pathogens with NMs with unique electrical, optical, catalytic, and pH indicators. We also discussed ideal tests that can rapidly, accurately, sensitively and selectively detect these bacteria.

Author details

Cemile Yilmaz[1], Cagla Celik[2], Nilay Ildiz[3], Esma Eryilmaz-Eren[4], Mehmet Akif Dündar[5], Uner Kayabas[4] and Ismail Ocsoy[1]*

1 Faculty of Pharmacy, Department of Analytical Chemistry, Erciyes University, Kayseri, Turkey

2 Harran University, Sanliurfa, Turkey

3 Bandirma Onyedi Eylul University, Balikesir, Turkey

4 University of Health Science, Kayseri City Training and Research Hospital, Kayseri, Turkey

5 Department of Pediatrics, Division of Pediatric Intensive Care, Kayseri City Training and Research Hospital, Health Sciences University, Kayseri, Turkey

*Address all correspondence to: ismailocsoy66@gmail.com

References

[1] American Academy of Pediatrics. *Staphylococcus aureus*. In: Kimberlin DW, Barnett ED, Lynfield R, Sawyer MH, editors. Red Book: 2021-2024 Report of the Committee on Infectious Diseases. 32nd ed. Itasca, IL: American Academy of Pediatrics; 2021. p. 678

[2] Tasneem U, Mehmood K, Majid M, Ullah SR, Andleeb S. Methicillin resistant *Staphylococcus aureus*: A brief review of virulence and resistance. JPMA. The Journal of the Pakistan Medical Association. 2022;**72**(3):509-515. DOI: 10.47391/jpma.0504

[3] Bai AD, Lo CK, Komorowski AS, Suresh M, Guo K, Garg A, et al. *Staphylococcus aureus* bacteraemia mortality: A systematic review and meta-analysis. Clinical Microbiology and Infection. 2022;**28**(8):1076-1084. DOI: 10.1016/j.cmi.2022.03.015

[4] Campbell AJ, Al Yazidi LS, Phuong LK, Leung C, Best EJ, Webb RH, et al. Pediatric *Staphylococcus aureus* bacteremia: Clinical spectrum and predictors of poor outcome. Clinical Infectious Diseases. 2022;**74**(4):604-613. DOI: 10.1093/cid/ciab510

[5] McMullan BJ, Campbell AJ, Blyth CC, McNeil JC, Montgomery CP, Tong SY, et al. Clinical management of *Staphylococcus aureus* bacteremia in neonates, children, and adolescents. Pediatrics. 2020;**146**(3):1-13. DOI: 10.1542/peds.2020-0134

[6] Southwick KL, Greenko J, Quinn MJ, Haley VB, Adams E, Lutterloh E. Methicillin-resistant *Staphylococcus aureus* (MRSA) clusters in neonatal intensive care units (NICUs) and other neonatal units in New York state (NYS), 2001 to 2017. American Journal of Infection Control. 2024;**52**(4):424-435. DOI: 10.1016/j.ajic.2023.09.015

[7] The Centers for Disease Control and Prevention. Recommendations for Prevention and Control of Infections in Neonatal Intensive Care Unit Patients: Staphylococcus aureus. 2020. Available from: https://www.cdc.gov/infection-control/hcp/nicu-saureus/? [Accessed: September 2, 2024]

[8] Batt CA. Materials science. Food pathogen detection. Science (New York, N.Y.). 2007;**316**(5831):1579-1580. DOI: 10.1126/science.114072

[9] Dykman L, Khlebtsov N. Gold nanoparticles in biomedical applications: Recent advances and perspectives. Chemical Society Reviews. 2012;**41**(6):2256-2282. DOI: 10.1039/C1CS15166E

[10] Saha K, Agasti SS, Kim C, Li X, Rotello VM. Gold nanoparticles in chemical and biological sensing. Chemical Reviews. 2012;**112**(5):2739-2779. DOI: 10.1021/cr2001178

[11] Zeng S, Yong KT, Roy I, Dinh XQ, Yu X, Luan F. A review on functionalized gold nanoparticles for biosensing applications. Plasmonics. 2011;**6**:491-506. DOI: 10.1007/s11468-011-9228-1

[12] Gao J, Liu D, Wang Z. Screening lectin-binding specificity of bacterium by lectin microarray with gold nanoparticle probes. Analytical Chemistry. 2010;**82**(22):9240-9247. DOI: 10.1021/ac1022309

[13] Madonna AJ, Basile F, Furlong E, Voorhees KJ. Detection of bacteria from biological mixtures using immunomagnetic separation combined

with matrix-assisted laser desorption/ionization time-of-flight mass spectrometry. Rapid Communications in Mass Spectrometry. 2001;**15**(13):1068-1074. DOI: 10.1002/rcm.344

[14] Yamaguchi N, Sasada M, Yamanaka M, Nasu M. Rapid detection of respiring *Escherichia coli* O157: H7 in apple juice, milk, and ground beef by flow cytometry. Cytometry Part A: the Journal of the International Society for Analytical Cytology. 2003;**54**(1):27-35. DOI: 10.1002/cyto.a.10045

[15] Glynn B, Lahiff S, Wernecke M, Barry T, Smith TJ, Maher M. Current and emerging molecular diagnostic technologies applicable to bacterial food safety. International Journal of Dairy Technology. 2006;**59**(2):126-139. DOI: 10.1111/j.1471-0307.2006.00253.x

[16] Celik C, Can Sezgin G, Kocabas UG, Gursoy S, Ildiz N, Tan W, et al. Novel anthocyanin-based colorimetric assay for the rapid, sensitive, and quantitative detection of *helicobacter pylori*. Analytical Chemistry. 2021;**93**(15):6246-6253. DOI: 0.1021/acs.analchem.1c00663

[17] Celik C, Ildiz N, Kaya MZ, Kilic AB, Ocsoy I. Preparation of natural indicator incorporated media and its logical use as a colorimetric biosensor for rapid and sensitive detection of methicillin-resistant *Staphylococcus aureus*. Analytica Chimica Acta. 2020;**1128**:80-89. DOI: 10.1016/j.aca.2020.06.005

[18] Celik C, Ildiz N, Sagiroglu P, Atalay MA, Yazici C, Ocsoy I. Preparation of nature inspired indicator based agar for detection and identification of MRSA and MRSE. Talanta. 2020;**219**:121292. DOI: 10.1016/j.talanta.2020.121292

[19] Celik C, Demir NY, Duman M, Ildiz N, Ocsoy I. Red cabbage extract-mediated colorimetric sensor for swift, sensitive and economic detection of urease-positive bacteria by naked eye and smartphone platform. Scientific Reports. 2023;**13**(1):2056. DOI: 10.1038/s41598-023-28604-1

[20] Celik C, Kalin G, Cetinkaya Z, Ildiz N, Ocsoy I. Recent advances in colorimetric tests for the detection of infectious diseases and antimicrobial resistance. Diagnostics. 2023;**13**(14):2427. DOI: 10.3390/diagnostics13142427

[21] Sezgin GC, Ocsoy I. Anthocyanin-rich black carrot (*Daucus carota ssp. sativus var. atrorubens* Alef.) and red cabbage (*Brassica oleracea*) extracts incorporated biosensor for colorimetric detection of *helicobacter pylori* with color image processing. Brazilian Journal of Microbiology. 2023;**54**(2):897-905. DOI: 10.1007/s42770-023-00989-1

[22] Sezgin GC, Tekin YE, Calim B, Celik C, Alrifai W, Temur N, et al. Development of a colorimetric urease test based on Au NPs capped with anthocyanin for the rapid detection of *helicobacter pylori* through multiple readouts. ChemistrySelect. 2023;**8**(27):e202300637. DOI: 10.1002/slct.202300637

[23] Shimada T, Ookubo K, Komuro N, Shimizu T, Uehara N. Blue-to-red chromatic sensor composed of gold nanoparticles conjugated with thermoresponsive copolymer for thiol sensing. Langmuir. 2007;**23**(22):11225-11232. DOI: 10.1021/la700664u

[24] Thaxton CS, Georganopoulou DG, Mirkin CA. Gold nanoparticle probes for the detection of nucleic acid targets. Clinica Chimica Acta. 2006;**363**(1-2):120-126. DOI: 10.1016/j.cccn.2005.05.042

[25] Schofield CL, Haines AH, Field RA, Russell DA. Silver and gold

glyconanoparticles for colorimetric bioassays. Langmuir. 2006;**22**(15):6707-6711. DOI: 10.1021/la060288r

[26] Shukoor MI, Altman MO, Han D, Bayrac AT, Ocsoy I, Zhu Z, et al. Aptamer-nanoparticle assembly for logic-based detection. ACS Applied Materials & Interfaces. 2012;**4**(6):3007-3011. DOI: 10.1021/am300374q

[27] Unal IS, Demirbas A, Onal I, Ildiz N, Ocsoy I. One step preparation of stable gold nanoparticle using red cabbage extracts under UV light and its catalytic activity. Journal of Photochemistry and Photobiology B: Biology. 2020;**204**:111800. DOI: 10.1016/j.jphotobiol.2020.111800

[28] Demirbas A, Büyükbezirci K, Celik C, Kislakci E, Karaagac Z, Gokturk E, et al. Synthesis of long-term stable gold nanoparticles benefiting from red raspberry (*Rubus idaeus*), strawberry (*Fragaria ananassa*), and blackberry (*Rubus fruticosus*) extracts–gold ion complexation and investigation of reaction conditions. ACS Omega. 2019;**4**(20):18637-18644. DOI: 10.1021/acsomega.9b02469

[29] McLamore ES, Convertino M, Ocsoy I, Vanegas DC, Taguchi M, Rong Y, et al. Biomimetic fractal nanometals as a transducer layer in electrochemical biosensing. In: Semiconductor-Based Sensors. Singapore: World Scientific Publishing Co. Pte. Ltd.; 2017. pp. 35-67. DOI: 10.1142/9789813146730_0002

[30] Howden BP, Giulieri SG, Wong Fok Lung T, Baines SL, Sharkey LK, Lee JY, et al. *Staphylococcus aureus* host interactions and adaptation. Nature Reviews Microbiology. 2023;**21**(6):380-395. DOI: 10.1038/s41579-023-00852-y

[31] Tong SY, Davis JS, Eichenberger E, Holland TL, Fowler VG Jr. *Staphylococcus aureus* infections: Epidemiology, pathophysiology, clinical manifestations, and management. Clinical Microbiology Reviews. 2015;**28**(3):603-661. DOI: 10.1128/cmr.00134-14

[32] Gherardi G. *Staphylococcus aureus* infection: Pathogenesis and antimicrobial resistance. International Journal of Molecular Sciences. 2023;**24**(9):8182. DOI: 10.3390/ijms24098182

[33] DeLeo FR, Diep BA, Otto M. Host defense and pathogenesis in Staphylococcus aureus infections. Infectious Disease Clinics of North America. 2009;**23**(1):17-34. DOI: 10.1016/j.idc.2008.10.003

[34] Renduchintala K, Nanjappa S, Ramsakal A, Greene J. Successful treatment of community-acquired methicillin-resistant *Staphylococcus aureus* necrotizing pneumonia in the setting of chronic graft-versus-host disease. Cureus. 2021;**13**(2):e13123. DOI: 10.7759/cureus.13123

[35] Rasul S, Farhat F, Asnake SA. Severe MRSA necrotizing pneumonia. Infection. 2013;**41**(1):299-300. DOI: 10.1007/s15010-012-0267-0

[36] Samia NI, Robicsek A, Heesterbeek H, Peterson LR. Methicillin-resistant *Staphylococcus aureus* nosocomial infection has a distinct epidemiological position and acts as a marker for overall hospital-acquired infection trends. Scientific Reports. 2022;**12**(1):17007. DOI: 10.1038/s41598-022-21300-6

[37] Rocha LEC, Singh V, Esch M, Lenaerts T, Liljeros F, Thorson A. Dynamic contact networks of patients and MRSA spread in hospitals. Scientific Reports. 2020;**10**(1):9336. DOI: 10.1038/s41598-020-66270-9

[38] Galar A, Weil AA, Dudzinski DM, Muñoz P, Siedner MJ. Methicillin-resistant *Staphylococcus aureus*

prosthetic valve endocarditis: Pathophysiology, epidemiology, clinical presentation, diagnosis, and management. Clinical Microbiology Reviews. 2019;**32**(2):e00041-e00018. DOI: 10.1128/cmr.00041-18

[39] Rupp M, Walter N, Bärtl S, Heyd R, Hitzenbichler F, Alt V. Fracture-related infection—Epidemiology, Etiology, diagnosis, prevention, and treatment. Deutsches Ärzteblatt International. 2024;**121**(1):17. DOI: 10.3238/arztebl.m2023.0233

[40] Monk EJ, Jones TP, Bongomin F, Kibone W, Nsubuga Y, Ssewante N, et al. Antimicrobial resistance in bacterial wound, skin, soft tissue and surgical site infections in central, eastern, southern and Western Africa: A systematic review and meta-analysis. PLOS Global Public Health. 2024;**4**(4):e0003077. DOI: 10.1371/journal.pgph.0003077

[41] Baker AW, Dicks KV, Durkin MJ, et al. Epidemiology of surgical site infection in a community hospital network. Infection Control & Hospital Epidemiology. 2016;**37**(5):519-526. DOI: 10.1017/ice.2016.13

[42] Zhu Z, Hu Z, Li S, Fang R, Ono HK, Hu D-L. Molecular characteristics and pathogenicity of *Staphylococcus aureus* exotoxins. International Journal of Molecular Sciences. 2024;**25**(1):395. DOI: 10.3390/ijms25010395

[43] Kanjilal S, Sater MR, Thayer M, Lagoudas GK, Kim S, Blainey PC, et al. Trends in antibiotic susceptibility in *Staphylococcus aureus* in Boston, Massachusetts, from 2000 to 2014. Journal of Clinical Microbiology. 2018;**56**(1):10-128. DOI: 10.1128/JCM.01160-17

[44] Aggarwal S, Jena S, Panda S, Sharma S, Dhawan B, Nath G, et al. Antibiotic susceptibility, virulence pattern, and typing of *Staphylococcus aureus* strains isolated from variety of infections in India. Frontiers in Microbiology. 2019;**10**:2763. DOI: 10.3389/fmicb.2019.02763

[45] Li J, Echevarria KL, Hughes DW, Cadena JA, Bowling JE, Lewis JS. Comparison of cefazolin versus oxacillin for treatment of complicated bacteremia caused by methicillin-susceptible *Staphylococcus aureus*. Antimicrobial Agents and Chemotherapy. 2014;**58**(9):5117-5124. DOI: 10.1128/AAC.02800-14

[46] Dutra KJ, Lazenby GB, Goje O, Soper DE. Cefazolin as the mainstay for antibiotic prophylaxis in patients with a penicillin allergy in obstetrics and gynecology. American Journal of Obstetrics and Gynecology. 2024;**231**(4):430-436. DOI: 10.1016/j.ajog.2024.03.019

[47] Bavaro DF, Belati A, Bussini L, Cento V, Diella L, Gatti M, et al. Safety and effectiveness of fifth generation cephalosporins for the treatment of methicillin-resistant *Staphylococcus aureus* bloodstream infections: A narrative review exploring past, present, and future. Expert Opinion on Drug Safety. 2024;**23**(1):9-36. DOI: 10.1080/14740338.2023.2299377

[48] Binda E, Marinelli F, Marcone GL. Old and new Glycopeptide antibiotics: Action and resistance. Antibiotics. 2014;**3**(4):572-594. DOI: 10.3390/antibiotics3040572

[49] Claeys KC, Zasowski EJ, Casapao AM, Lagnf AM, Nagel JL, Nguyen CT, et al. Daptomycin improves outcomes regardless of vancomycin MIC in a propensity-matched analysis of methicillin-resistant *Staphylococcus aureus* bloodstream infections. Antimicrobial Agents and

Chemotherapy. 2016;**60**(10):5841-5848. DOI: 10.1128/AAC.00227-16

[50] Schweizer ML, Richardson K, Vaughan Sarrazin MS, Goto M, Livorsi DJ, Nair R, et al. Comparative effectiveness of switching to daptomycin versus remaining on vancomycin among patients with methicillin-resistant *Staphylococcus aureus* (MRSA) bloodstream infections. Clinical Infectious Diseases. 2021;**72**(Supplement. 1):S68-S73. DOI: 10.1093/cid/ciaa1572

[51] Guskey MT, Tsuji BT. A comparative review of the lipoglycopeptides: Oritavancin, dalbavancin, and telavancin. Pharmacotherapy. 2010;**30**(1):80-94. DOI: 10.1592/phco.30.1.80

[52] Moellering RC Jr. Linezolid: The first oxazolidinone antimicrobial. Annals of Internal Medicine. 2003;**139**(10):864. DOI: 10.7326/0003-4819-138-2-200301210-00015

[53] Kaushik A, Kest H, Sood M, Steussy BW, Thieman C, Gupta S. Biofilm producing methicillin-resistant *Staphylococcus aureus* (MRSA) infections in humans: Clinical implications and management. Pathogens. 2024;**13**(1):76. DOI: 10.3390/pathogens13010076

[54] Sanchini A. Recent developments in phenotypic and molecular diagnostic methods for antimicrobial resistance detection in *Staphylococcus aureus*: A narrative review. Diagnostics. 2022;**12**(1):208. DOI: 10.3390/diagnostics12010208

[55] Kim JK, Yun HY, Kim JS, Kim W, Lee CS, Kim BG, et al. Development of fluorescence-linked immunosorbent assay for rapid detection of *Staphylococcus aureus*. Applied Microbiology and Biotechnology. 2024;**108**(1):2. DOI: 10.1007/s00253-023-12836-2. Epub 2023 Dec 28

[56] Duan R, Wang P. Rapid and simple approaches for diagnosis of in bloodstream infections. Polish Journal of Microbiology. 2022;**71**(4):481-489. DOI: 10.33073/pjm-2022-050

[57] Gill AA, Singh S, Thapliyal N, Karpoormath R. Nanomaterial-based optical and electrochemical techniques for detection of methicillin-resistant *Staphylococcus aureus*: A review. Microchimica Acta. 2019;**186**:1-9. DOI: 10.1007/s00604-018-3186-7

[58] Alberti G, Zanoni C, Magnaghi LR, Biesuz R. Gold and silver nanoparticle-based colorimetric sensors: New trends and applications. Chem. 2021;**9**(11):305. DOI: 10.3390/chemosensors9110305

[59] Shahbazi R, Salouti M, Amini B, Jalilvand A, Naderlou E, Amini A, et al. Highly selective and sensitive detection of *Staphylococcus aureus* with gold nanoparticle-based core-shell nano biosensor. Molecular and Cellular Probes. 2018;**41**:8-13. DOI: 10.1016/j.mcp.2018.07.004

[60] Khan MQ, Khan J, Alvi MA, Nawaz H, Fahad M, Umar M. Nanomaterial-based sensors for microbe detection: A review. Discover Nano. 2024;**19**(1):120. DOI: 10.1186/s11671-024-04065-x

[61] Choi Y, Hwang JH, Lee SY. Recent trends in nanomaterials-based colorimetric detection of pathogenic bacteria and viruses. Small Methods. 2018;**2**(4):1700351. DOI: 10.1002/smtd.201700351

[62] Najafabad MB, Rastin SJ, Taghvaei F, Khiyavi AA. A review on applications of gold nanoparticles-based biosensor for pathogen detection. Advances in

Natural Sciences: Nanoscience and Nanotechnology. 2022;**13**(3):033002. DOI: 10.1088/2043-6262/ac79ae

[63] Yuan J, Wu S, Duan N, Ma X, Xia Y, Chen J, et al. A sensitive gold nanoparticle-based colorimetric aptasensor for *Staphylococcus aureus*. Talanta. 2014;**127**:163-168. DOI: 10.1016/j.talanta.2014.04.013

[64] Liu A, Zhang Y, Chen W, Wang X, Chen F. Gold nanoparticle-based colorimetric detection of staphylococcal enterotoxin B using ssDNA aptamers. European Food Research and Technology. 2013;**237**:323-329. DOI: 10.1007/s00217-013-1995-9

[65] Zhang Y, Chen Y, Han D, Ocsoy I, Tan W. Aptamers selected by cell-SELEX for application in cancer studies. Bioanalysis. 2010;**2**(5):907-918. DOI: 10.4155/bio.10.46

[66] Arslan Ocsoy M, Yusufbeyoglu S, Ildiz N, Ulgen A, Ocsoy I. DNA aptamer-conjugated magnetic graphene oxide for pathogenic bacteria aggregation: Selective and enhanced photothermal therapy for effective and rapid killing. ACS Omega. 2021;**6**(31):20637-20643. DOI: 10.1021/acsomega.1c02832

[67] Turek D, Van Simaeys D, Johnson J, Ocsoy I, Tan W. Molecular recognition of live methicillin-resistant *Staphylococcus aureus* cells using DNA aptamers. World Journal of Translational Medicine. 2013;**2**(3):67-74. DOI: 10.5528/wjtm.v2.i3.67

[68] Ocsoy I, Yusufbeyoglu S, Yılmaz V, McLamore ES, Ildız N, Ülgen A. DNA aptamer functionalized gold nanostructures for molecular recognition and photothermal inactivation of methicillin-resistant *Staphylococcus aureus*. Colloids and Surfaces B: Biointerfaces. 2017;**159**:16-22. DOI: 10.1016/j.colsurfb.2017.07.056

[69] Wang J, Gao J, Liu D, Han D, Wang Z. Phenylboronic acid functionalized gold nanoparticles for highly sensitive detection of *Staphylococcus aureus*. Nanoscale. 2012;**4**(2):451-454. DOI: 10.1039/C2NR11657J

[70] Pilecky M, Schildberger A, Knabl L, Orth-Höller D, Weber V. Influence of antibiotic treatment on the detection of S. Aureus in whole blood following pathogen enrichment. BMC Microbiology. 2019;**19**:1-9. DOI: 10.1186/s12866-019-1559-7

[71] dos Santos SR, Corrêa CR, de Barros AL, Serakides R, Fernandes SO, Cardoso VN, et al. Identification of Staphylococcus aureus infection by aptamers directly radiolabeled with technetium-99m. Nuclear Medicine and Biology. 2015;**42**(3):292-298. DOI: 10.1016/j.nucmedbio.2014.12.002

[72] Roth-Konforti M, Green O, Hupfeld M, Fieseler L, Heinrich N, Ihssen J, et al. Ultrasensitive detection of *salmonella* and *listeria monocytogenes* by small-molecule chemiluminescence probes. Angewandte Chemie. 2019;**131**(30):10469-10475. DOI: 10.1002/ange.201904719

[73] Adkins JA, Boehle K, Friend C, Chamberlain B, Bisha B, Henry CS. Colorimetric and electrochemical bacteria detection using printed paper-and transparency-based analytic devices. Analytical Chemistry. 2017;**89**(6):3613-3621. DOI: 10.1021/acs.analchem.6b05009

[74] Xu D, Wu L, Yao H, Zhao L. Catalase-like nanozymes: Classification, catalytic mechanisms, and their applications. Small. 2022;**18**(37):2203400. DOI: 10.1002/smll.202203400

[75] Hosseini M. Fast and selective whole cell detection of *Staphylococcus*

aureus bacteria in food samples by paper based colorimetric nanobiosensor using peroxidase-like catalytic activity of DNA-Au/Pt bimetallic nanoclusters. Microchemical Journal. 2020;**159**:105475. DOI: 10.1016/j.microc.2020.105475

[76] Yao S, Li J, Pang B, Wang X, Shi Y, Song X, et al. Colorimetric immunoassay for rapid detection of *Staphylococcus aureus* based on etching-enhanced peroxidase-like catalytic activity of gold nanoparticles. Microchimica Acta. 2020;**187**:1-8. DOI: 10.1007/s00604-020-04473-7

[77] Zhang H, Yao S, Song X, Xu K, Wang J, Li J, et al. One-step colorimetric detection of *Staphylococcus aureus* based on target-induced shielding against the peroxidase mimicking activity of aptamer-functionalized gold-coated iron oxide nanocomposites. Talanta. 2021;**232**:122448. DOI: 10.1016/j.talanta.2021.122448

[78] Gao B, Ding Y, Cai Z, Wu S, Wang J, Ling N, et al. Dual-recognition colorimetric platform based on porous Au@ Pt nanozymes for highly sensitive washing-free detection of *Staphylococcus aureus*. Microchimica Acta. 2024;**191**(7):438. DOI: 10.1007/s00604-024-06460-8

[79] Liu Y, Sun M, Qiao W, Cong S, Zhang Y, Wang L, et al. Multicolor colorimetric visual detection of *Staphylococcus aureus* based on Fe3O4–Ag–MnO2 composites nano-oxidative mimetic enzyme. Analytica Chimica Acta. 2023;**1239**:340654. DOI: 10.1016/j.aca.2022.340654

[80] Duan B, Li B, Ma L, Niu X, Yang Y, Zhang X. Colorimetric detection of *Staphylococcus aureus* based on self-linkable and hollow organic-inorganic nanocomposites as light-driven oxidase-like nanozyme for cascade signal amplification. Sensors and Actuators B: Chemical. 2024;**409**:135547. DOI: 10.1016/j.snb.2024.135547

[81] Mahadeva SK, Walus K, Stoeber B. Paper as a platform for sensing applications and other devices: A review. ACS Applied Materials & Interfaces. 2015;**7**(16):8345-8362. DOI: 10.1021/acsami.5b00373

[82] Mao K, Min X, Zhang H, Zhang K, Cao H, Guo Y, et al. Based microfluidics for rapid diagnostics and drug delivery. Journal of Controlled Release. 2020;**322**:187-199. DOI: 10.1016/j.jconrel.2020.03.010

[83] Pan Y, Mao K, Hui Q, Wang B, Cooper J, Yang Z. Based devices for rapid diagnosis and wastewater surveillance. TrAC Trends in Analytical Chemistry. 2022;**157**:116760. DOI: 10.1016/j.trac.2022.116760

[84] Terry SC, Jerman JH, Angell JB. A gas chromatographic air analyzer fabricated on a silicon wafer. IEEE Transactions on Electron Devices. 1979;**26**(12):1880-1886. DOI: 10.1109/T-ED.1979.19791

[85] Martinez AW, Phillips ST, Butte MJ, Whitesides GM. Patterned paper as a platform for inexpensive, low-volume, portable bioassays. Angewandte Chemie. 2007;**119**(8):1340-1342. DOI: 10.1002/anie.200603817

[86] Reboud J, Xu G, Garrett A, Adriko M, Yang Z, Tukahebwa EM, et al. Based microfluidics for DNA diagnostics of malaria in low resource underserved rural communities. National Academy of Sciences of the United States of America. 2019;**116**(11):4834-4842. DOI: 10.1073/pnas.1812296116

[87] Yang Z, Xu G, Reboud J, Ali SA, Kaur G, McGiven J, et al. Rapid veterinary diagnosis of bovine

reproductive infectious diseases from semen using paper-origami DNA microfluidics. ACS Sensors. 2018;**3**(2):403-409. DOI: 10.1021/acssensors.7b00825

[88] Ratnarathorn N, Chailapakul O, Henry CS, Dungchai W. Simple silver nanoparticle colorimetric sensing for copper by paper-based devices. Talanta. 2012;**99**:552-557. DOI: 10.1016/j.talanta.2012.06.033

[89] Somvanshi SB, Ulloa AM, Zhao M, Liang Q, Barui AK, Lucas A, et al. Microfluidic paper-based aptasensor devices for multiplexed detection of pathogenic bacteria. Biosensors and Bioelectronics. 2022;**207**:114214. DOI: 10.1016/j.bios.2022.114214

[90] Suea-Ngam A, Choopara I, Li S, Schmelcher M, Somboonna N, Howes PD, et al. In situ nucleic acid amplification and ultrasensitive colorimetric readout in a paper-based analytical device using silver Nanoplates. Advanced Healthcare Materials. 2021;**10**(7):2001755. DOI: 10.1002/adhm.202001755, 2001755

[91] Dungchai W, Chailapakul O, Henry CS. Electrochemical detection for paper-based microfluidics. Analytical chemistry. 2009;**81**(14):5821-5826. DOI: 10.1021/ac9007573

[92] Jiang H, Yang J, Wan K, Jiang D, Jin C. Miniaturized paper-supported 3D cell-based electrochemical sensor for bacterial lipopolysaccharide detection. ACS Sensors. 2020;**5**(5):1325-1335. DOI: 10.1021/acssensors.9b02508

[93] Mandal PK, Biswas AK, Choi K, Pal UK. Methods for rapid detection of foodborne pathogens: An overview. American Journal of Food Technology. 2011;**6**(2):87-102. DOI: 10.3923/ajft.2011.87.102

[94] Lu C, Gao X, Chen Y, Ren J, Liu C. Aptamer-based lateral flow test strip for the simultaneous detection of *salmonella typhimurium, Escherichia coli* O157: H7 and *Staphylococcus aureus*. Analytical Letters. 2020;**53**(4):646-659. DOI: 10.1080/00032719.2019.1663528

[95] Guo J, Zhong Z, Li Y, Liu Y, Wang R, Ju H. "Three-in-one" SERS adhesive tape for rapid sampling, release, and detection of wound infectious pathogens. ACS applied Materials & Interfaces. 2019;**11**(40):36399-36408. DOI: 10.1021/ACSAMI.9B12823

[96] Wang CH, Wu JJ, Lee GB. Screening of highly-specific aptamers and their applications in paper-based microfluidic chips for rapid diagnosis of multiple bacteria. Sensors and Actuators B: Chemical. 2019;**284**:395-402. DOI: 10.1016/J.SNB.2018.12.112

[97] Suaifan GA, Alhogail S, Zourob M. Rapid and low-cost biosensor for the detection of *Staphylococcus aureus*. Biosensors and Bioelectronics. 2017;**90**:230-237. DOI: 10.1016/j.bios.2016.11.047

[98] Sheini A. A point-of-care testing sensor based on fluorescent nanoclusters for rapid detection of septicemia in children. Sensors and Actuators B: Chemical. 2021;**328**:129029. DOI: 10.1016/j.snb.2020.129029

[99] Sekar V, Santhanam A, Arunkumar P. A low-cost paper and solution based colorimetric detection of bacteria using glucose-functionalized gold nanoparticles. Journal of Water Process Engineering. 2024;**59**:105102. DOI: 10.1016/j.jwpe.2024.105102

[100] Albashir D, Lu H, Gouda M, Acharya DR, Danhassan UA, Bakur A, et al. A novel polydiacetylene-functionalized fibrinogen paper-based

biosensor for on-spot and rapid detection of *Staphylococcus aureus*. Food Chemistry. 2024;**458**:140291. DOI: 10.1016/j.foodchem.2024.140291

[101] Lee S, Reo SH, Kim S, Kim S, Lee ES, Cha BS, et al. Colorimetric detection of *Staphylococcus aureus* based on direct loop-mediated isothermal amplification in combination with lateral flow assay. BioChip Journal. 2024;**18**(1):85-92. DOI: 10.1007/s13206-023-00130-2

Chapter 4

Detection and Typing of *Staphylococcus aureus* Strains in Pediatric Population of Mexico City

Anaid Bustos-Hamdan, Samuel González García, Juan Antonio Guzmán Salgado, Aída Hamdan-Partida and Jaime Bustos-Martínez

Abstract

Staphylococcus aureus is one of the main bacteria that infect humans. The pediatric population is susceptible to this microorganism; in Mexico there are not enough epidemiological studies on this subject, so the objective of this work was to detect and typify *S. aureus* strains in an apparently healthy pediatric population of daycare centers and schools. Nasal and pharyngeal exudates were collected to determine the presence of these bacteria and typed as HA-MRSA or CA-MRSA strains by determining SCC*mec*, *mecA* gene, Panton-Valentine leucocidin (PVL), phenol-soluble modulin (*psm*), and *spa*-type. It was found that 62.55% of the population were carriers of *S. aureus*, with a higher percentage in the pharynx and in children older than 4 years of age. A total of 7.04% were carriers of MRSA strains, of which 14.64% were HA-MRSA strains and 85.36% were CA-MRSA strains. The strains showed resistance to several antibiotics. About 20% of the MRSA strains had PVL and *psm* genes. The strains presented a great variety of *spa*-types. A high number of *S. aureus* carriers were found in the pediatric population studied, with the presence of CA-MRSA strains, so surveillance and decolonization programs should be established.

Keywords: *Staphylococcus aureus*, pediatric population, CA-MRSA, HA-MRSA, *spa*-type, antibiotic resistance

1. Introduction

Staphylococcus aureus is a bacterium with the shape of cocci grouped in clusters, Gram positive, facultative anaerobic, nonmotile, ferments mannitol and is halophilic, and is positive to the catalase, oxidase and coagulase tests. It is a commensal bacterium that can become pathogenic because it possesses virulence factors that allow it to survive innate immune mechanisms when entering humans, among which are adhesins that allow it to anchor to host cells to begin colonization, exoenzymes that degrade molecular components of tissues, superantigens and toxins, it can also synthesize polysaccharides associated with surfaces and capsule to protect itself, among many other factors that allow it to persist and resist multiple antibiotics [1, 2].

The most pathogenic *S. aureus* strains are those with methicillin resistance, methicillin-resistant *Staphylococcus aureus* (MRSA), which is included in the ESKAPE group (*Enterococcus faecium*, *S. aureus*, *Klebsiella pneumoniae*, *Acinetobacter baumannii*, *Pseudomonas aeruginosa* y *Enterobacter* spp), of multidrug-resistant bacteria [1], this bacterium has generated a high mortality rate worldwide and one of the most affected populations is the pediatric population [3]. Another important strain is methicillin-sensitive *Staphylococcus aureus* (MSSA), which has gained more ground at the hospital level [4]. MRSA strains can be divided into three main types, corresponding to community-acquired methicillin-resistant *S. aureus* (CA-MRSA), hospital-acquired (HA-MRSA) and livestock-associated (LA-MRSA) [1]. In reports from the 1960s, strains isolated at the hospital level (HA-MRSA) were observed for the first time, and in the 1990s the first cases of infections at the community level (CA-MRSA) were reported [5, 6].

Previously it was believed that infections produced by MRSA strains in the hospital were the most serious, however, nowadays community infections are also behaving in a serious way including in the pediatric population. This problem has to do in part with the indiscriminate use of antibiotics, which has generated a condition of multi-resistance to antibiotics in strains of *S. aureus*, placing it on the WHO list as a priority pathogen resistant to antibiotics [5–7].

The risk of infection by *S. aureus*, especially MRSA strains, increases among different susceptible populations such as children, the elderly, athletes, overcrowded living conditions, the military, people who use injectable drugs, immunodeficient people, and even people who frequent hospital centers [5, 6]. This risk of infection usually occurs due to increased exposure to the bacteria and decreased defense mechanisms in different at-risk populations [5, 7].

Colonization by this bacterium is a risk factor for triggering invasive infections in hospitals and communities [5–7]. Colonization tends to be mainly at the nasal and pharyngeal level where it predisposes to suffer from infections ranging from mild to complicated [8]. As has been reported in previous studies, there is a colonization by *S. aureus* with a different percentage according to the colonized site. *S. aureus* colonization at the level of the nose has been reported in 20–40% of the general population [5], while in the pharynx colonization ranges from 4 to 64% [8].

Currently, it is known that there are multiple factors to trigger colonization, for example, the airway, food, skin-to-skin contact, age, especially children and older adults, immunocompromised persons, livestock farmers. Up to 30% of people are colonized by *S. aureus* permanently and 30% are usually colonized intermittently, and 2–10% are colonized with MRSA strains [7, 9].

As it has been reported worldwide about one-third of the population is colonized by *S. aureus*, this allows it to be an important factor producing infections in the different stages of life [7]. *S. aureus* is an agent with a high prevalence rate either at the hospital level, mainly with MRSA strains, or at the community level with MSSA and MRSA strains [7, 9].

Infections caused by *S. aureus* have increased in recent years, including in the pediatric population [7, 9, 10]. Studies show that *S. aureus* is the main cause of pediatric infections and soft tissue infections in children, and it is also the second cause of death due to neonatal sepsis [10, 11].

Pediatric *S. aureus* infections can range from mild to life-threatening infections such as necrotizing fasciitis, bacteremia, osteomyelitis and endocarditis, resulting in a high mortality of up to 22–66% [7, 10].

There are risk factors related to pediatric colonization and infection, among the main pediatric factors that have been related are age, children 12 months old, prematurity, low birth weight (<1500 g), asthma and eczema [4, 12].

However, the epidemiology of pediatric *S. aureus* infections is highly variable worldwide, which varies depending on the countries studied; a percentage of up to 48% has been reported in the United States [3]. In the case of MSSA strains, it has been described that they can cause an incidence of infections up to 2.2% higher than infections caused by MRSA strains [4, 7, 11]. Currently, there has been an increase in the number of cases in the pediatric population at the level of community infections with CA-MRSA strains, but HA-MRSA strains should not be overlooked [3]. Therefore, it is essential to have knowledge of the epidemiology of *S. aureus*, the type of strains, their characteristics and virulence factors that may be involved in the infection and their resistance to antibiotics, this information is crucial in the diagnosis and timely treatment at the pediatric level, in order to avoid further morbidity and mortality [3].

In Mexico, there are not enough epidemiological studies on the prevalence of *S. aureus* in the pediatric population, so the objective of this study was to determine and typify the presence of this bacterium in the pediatric population of Mexico City.

2. Methods

2.1 Sampling

Pharyngeal and nasal swabs were collected from 582 apparently healthy children and adolescents aged 6 months to 18 years from daycare centers and schools in Mexico City between 2013 and 2019. Informed consent was requested for sample collection and parental consent was requested for minors. Nasal sampling was performed by inserting a sterile swab into both nostrils, and pharyngeal sampling was performed with another swab by gently scraping the oropharynx. Both swabs were stored and transported in separate tubes with trypticase soy broth (TSB) at room temperature until reaching the laboratory, where they were incubated at 37°C for 24 h, after which time they were inoculated in salt and mannitol agar dishes by the cross-stretch method and incubated for 24 h at 37°C.

2.2 Identification of *Staphylococcus aureus*

All strains that grew on mannitol salt agar as circular yellow colonies measuring 2–3 mm in diameter and that turned the color of the agar yellow, and that the coagulase test was positive, were considered as *S. aureus*, if any strain presented inconclusive results, DNA was extracted using the DNA Wizard Genomic Extraction Kit, to perform a PCR of the 16S rRNA gene [13] and subsequent sequencing at Macrogen Korea, the sequences were identified using nBLAST.

2.3 Antibiogram

The antibiogram test was performed on all *S. aureus* strains using the Kirby-Bauer method according to CLSI guidelines [14], strains were grown in TSB at 37°C overnight, in a tube with sterile Mueller-Hinton broth the bacterial suspension was adjusted to a concentration of 0.5 McFarland units using a Densimat (bioMériux, France), then a sterile swab was dipped in the bacterial suspension to massively seed a Mueller-Hinton agar plate, Gram-positive polydisks (PBM, Mexico) were used, for the antibiotics: ciprofloxacin (CIP), fosfomycin (FO), trimethoprim-sulfamethoxazole (TSX), penicillin (P), vancomycin (VA), tetracycline (TE), Erythromycin (E), oxacillin (OX), macrolides (MAC), clindamycin (CC), gentamicin (GM) and cephalothin (CF).

2.4 Identification of MRSA strains

The minimum inhibitory concentration (MIC) test for oxacillin was performed according to CLSI guidelines [14], MRSA strains were considered to be those that grew at concentrations of ≥4 μg/mL, using *S. aureus* strains ATCC 43300 and ATCC 29213 as positive and negative controls, respectively. The presence of the *mecA* gene was also determined by PCR following the methodology previously described [15, 16].

For the typing of MRSA strains, the identification of the staphylococcal cassette chromosome (SCC*mec*) was performed by multiplex PCR [15] using the primers CIF2 F2, CIF2 R2, MECI P2, MECI P3, RIF5 F10 and FIF5 R13, at a final concentration of 400 nM, in addition to the primers DCS F2, DCS R2, MECA P4 and MECA P7 at a final concentration of 800 nM, and the primers KDP F1, KDP R1, RIF4 F3 and RIF4 R9 at a final concentration of 200 nM (**Table 1**). The thermocycling conditions were: initial denaturation for 4 minutes at 94°C; followed by 30 cycles of 94°C for 30 seconds, 53°C for 30 seconds and 72°C for 1 minute, plus a final extension of 4 minutes at 72°C, ending by maintaining the temperature at 4°C. In addition, another multiplex PCR was performed with the conditions reported by Boye et al. in 2007 [16], using the primers β, α-3 (0.2 μM), ccrCF, ccrCR (0.25 μM), 1272F1, 1272R1 (0.08 μM) and 5RmecA and 5R431 (0.1 μM) (**Table 1**), with the following thermocycling conditions: initial denaturation at 94°C for 4 minutes, followed by 30 cycles of 30 seconds at 94°C, 30 seconds at 55°C and 1 minute at 72°C, with a final extension at 72°C for 4 minutes. *S. aureus* strains BAA-44, BAA-41, BAA-39, NRS 643 and NRS 745 were used as positive controls for SCC*mec* cassettes I, II, III, IV and V, respectively.

The presence of *lukS-PV/lukF-PV* genes of Panton-Valentine leukocidin (PVL) was amplified by end-point PCR using the primers reported by Lina et al. [17] (**Table 1**), with a thermocycling of 5 minutes of initial denaturation at 94°C, followed by 30 cycles of 30 seconds at 94°C, 55°C 30 seconds, and one minute of extension at 72°C, using as a positive control the strain of *S. aureus* BAA-1680, the gene of the phenol soluble modulin (*psm*) was also amplified by end-point PCR following the methodology and primers published by Mehlin et al. [18] (**Table 1**), with the thermocycling conditions of: 4 minutes at 94°C of initial denaturation, followed by 35 cycles of 15 s at 94°C, 15 s at 55°C and 90 s at 72°C, with a final extension at 72°C for 9.5 minutes.

Typing of *S. aureus* (*spa*-typing) was obtained by amplifying the *spa* gene through PCR with the following thermocycling conditions: initial denaturation at 80°C for 5 minutes, followed by 35 cycles of 94°C 45 s, 60°C 45 s, 72°C 90 s, plus 10 minutes of final extension at 72°C, using the primers published by Shopsin et al. [19] (**Table 1**), and the *S. aureus* strain ATCC 43300 as a positive control, and subsequently sequencing the amplicons in MacroGen (Korea). The *spa*-types were assigned using the SPA Searcher (http://seqtools.com) and Ridom GmbH (http://spaserver.ridom.de/) website. Community-acquired strains (CA-MRSA) strains were considered as CA-MRSA strains if they had SCC*mec* IV, IVa or V and could have the PVL gene, and hospital-acquired strains (HA-MRSA) were typed as HA-MRSA strains if they had SCC*mec* I, II or III [20].

Genes	Primers	Sequence (5′-3′)	Amplicon (bp)	Reference
SCC*mec*	CICF F2 CIF2 R2	TTCGAGTTGCTGATGAAGAAGG ATTTACCACAAGGACTACCAGC	495	[15]
	KDP F1 KDP R1	AATCATCTGCCATTGGTGATGC CGAATGAAGTGAAAGAAAGTGG	284	
	MECI P2 MECI P3	ATCAAGACTTGCATTCAGGC GCGGTTTCAATTCACTTGTC	209	
	DCS F2 DCS R1	CATCCTATGATAGCTTGGTC CTAAATCATAGCCATGACCG	342	
	RIF4 F3 RIF4 R9	GTGATTGTTCGAGATATGTGG CGCTTTATCTGTATCTATCGC	243	
mecA	MECA P4 MECA P7	TCCAGATTACAACTTCACCAGG CCACTTCATATCTTGTAACG	162	[15]
SCC*mec*	β α-3	ATTGCCTTGATAATAGCCYTCT TAAAGGCATCAATGCACAAACACT	937	[16]
	ccrCF ccrCR	CGTCTATTACAAGATGTTAAGGATAAT CCTTTATAGACTGGATTATTCAAAATAT	518	
	1272F1 1272R1	GCCACTCATAACATATGGAA CATCCGAGTGAAACCCAAA	415	
	5RmecA 5R431	TATACCAAACCCGACAACTAC CGGCTACAGTGATAACATCC	359	
PVL	*luk*-PV-F *luk*-PV-R	GCATCAASTGTATTGGATAGCAAAAGC ATCATTAGGTAAAATGTCTGGACATGATCCA	433	[17]
psm	PSMa	TCCTTCCTTTCGATGTCGTT CCATCTTTTACGATGGTGGTTT	221	[18]
spa	spa-1113 F spa-1514 R	TAAAGACGATCCTTCGGTGAGC CAGCAGTAGTGCCGTTTGCTT	443	[19]

bp: base pairs.

Table 1.
Primers used in the identification and typing of S. aureus *strains.*

All PCR reactions were performed using the commercial PCR Master Mix 2X kit (Promega, USA) in the MyClycer thermal cycler (BioRad, USA). PCR products were identified by performing 1% agarose gel electrophoresis (BioRad) in 0.5X Tris Borate EDTA buffer (TBE, BioRad), the agar gel was placed in an ethidium bromide solution (0.5 μg/mL) and developed in a UV light transilluminator (SYNGENE).

2.5 Statistical analysis

The chi-square test and Fischer's F test were performed considering values with a statistical difference of $p < 0.05$ with SPSS software version 25.0. (IBM, NY, USA).

3. Results

3.1 *S. aureus* carriers

We analyzed 317 women (54.46%) and 265 men (45.54%), with a mean age of 9.38 years (±5.13), finding that 62.55% (364) are *S. aureus* carriers, of which 159 (27.31%) are carriers in both sites, 125 (21.47%) are exclusive pharynx carriers and 80 (13.74%) are exclusive carriers in the nose. Thus, pharynx carriers are more than nose carriers. In addition, 218 (37.45%) were found not to be *S. aureus* carriers (**Table 2**). Women presented a slightly higher percentage of carriers than men (35.33% vs. 27.31%), the greatest significant difference being found in exclusive nose carriers where in women it was 10.8% vs. 2.92% in men (**Table 2**). In addition, a total of 523 *S. aureus* strains were isolated, of which 284 were found in the pharynx (54.30%) and 239 in the nose (45.70%).

Carriers were analyzed by age group. Group 1: 141 individuals aged 1–3 years; Group 2: 143 individuals aged 4–6 years; Group 3: 180 individuals aged 7–9 years; Group 4: 100 individuals aged 10–12 years; Group 5: 7 individuals aged 13–15 years and Group 6: 111 individuals aged 16–18 years. In these groups, the percentage of *S. aureus* carriers found were 9.75%; 56.64%; 71.11% ($p < 0.05$ with respect to carriers 1–3, years); 82% ($p < 0.01$ with respect to carriers 1–3, years); 42.85% and 59.45%, respectively (**Figure 1**).

3.2 Antibiotic resistance and identification of MSSA and MRSA strains of *S. aureus*

The antibiotic to which the isolated *S. aureus* strains show the greatest resistance is penicillin (87% overall resistance, 89% in nasal strains and 84% in pharyngeal

	Carriers and non-carriers of *S. aureus*				
	Non-carriers	**Carriers**	**Both sites**	**Pharynx**	**Nose**
N = 582	218 (37.45%)	364 (62.55%)*	159 (27.31%)	125 (21.47%)	80 (13.74%)
Women (n = 317) 54.46%	112 (19.14%)	205 (35.22%)	83 (14.26%)	59 (10.13%)	63 (10.80%)**
Men (n = 265) 45.54%	106 (18.20%)	159 (27.31%)	76 (13.05%)	66 (11.34%)	17 (2.92%)

*When comparing non-carrier vs. carrier: * $p < 0.05$; when comparing isolated female vs. male nasal carriers: ** $p < 0.01$.*

Table 2.
Carriers of S. aureus *in the pediatric population analyzed.*

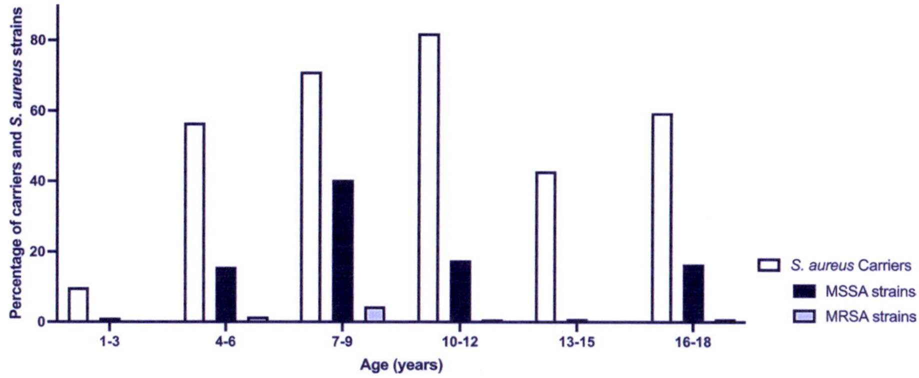

Figure 1.
Percentage of S. aureus *carriers and MSSA and MRSA strains isolated by age group.*

strains), followed by erythromycin (34% overall resistance, 32% in pharyngeal strains and 31% in nasal strains), and in third place clindamycin and tetracycline (with an overall resistance of 14%, 17% in the nose and 13% in the pharynx). Other antibiotics such as cephalothin, macrolides, ciprofloxacin, trimethoprim-sulfamethoxazole and fosfomycin showed similar resistance percentages (between 8 and 12% resistance). In the case of gentamicin and oxacillin, less than 8% of the isolated strains showed resistance and no strain was resistant to vancomycin (**Figure 2**).

Regarding methicillin resistance, it was found that 482 (92.16%) strains were MSSA ($p < 0.0001$), of which 209 (39.96%) were found in nose and 273 (52.20%) in pharynx (**Figure 3**). Regarding gender, 278 strains were isolated from males (57.67%) and 204 were isolated from females (42.33%) ($p > 0.05$). When analyzed by age group, 6 MSSA strains were found in 1–3-year-olds (1.14%), 82 in the 4–6-year-old group (15.67%), 211 in the 7–9-year-olds (40.34%, $p < 0.01$), 92 in the 10–12 year

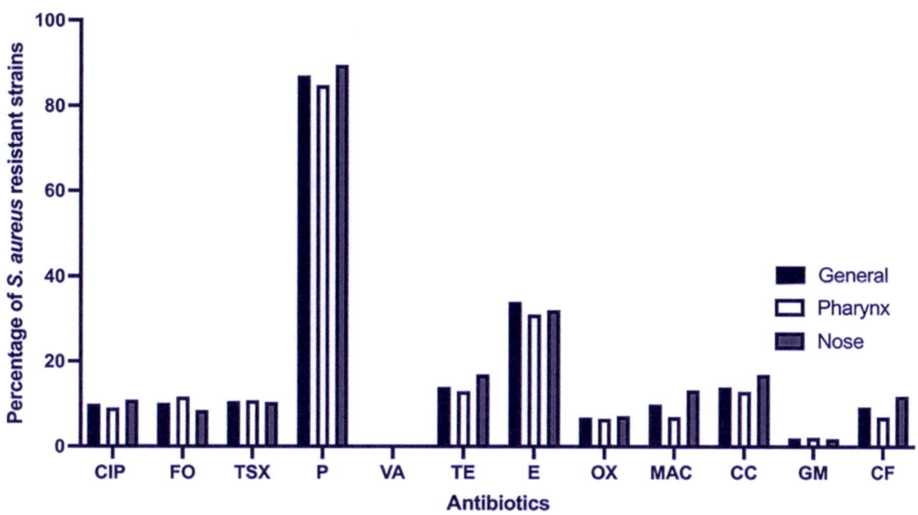

Figure 2.
Percentage of S. aureus *strains resistant to antibiotics. CIP: ciprofloxacin, FO: fosfomycin. TSX: trimethoprim-sulfamethoxazole, P: penicillin, VA: vancomycin, TE: tetracycline, E: erythromycin, OX: oxacillin, MAC: macrolides, CC: clindamycin, GM: gentamicin, and CF: cephalothin.*

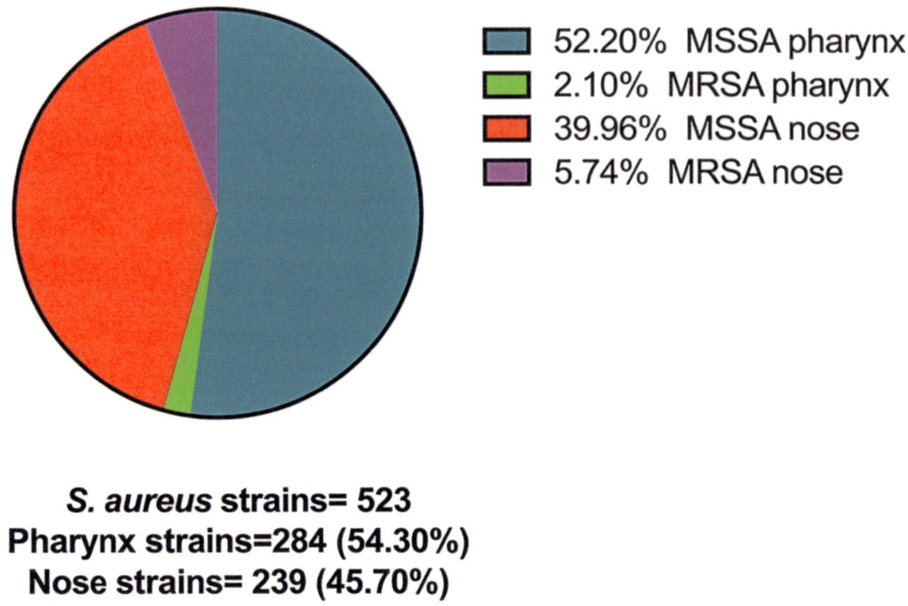

Figure 3.
MSSA and MRSA strains isolated from pharynx and nose.

old group (17.59%), 5 strains in the 13–15-year-old group (0.95%) and 86 MSSA strains in the 16–18-year-old group (16.44%) (**Figure 1**).

It was found that 7.04% of the studied population were carriers of MRSA strains. Forty-one MRSA strains were isolated representing 7.84% of the total number of *S. aureus* strains, of which 11 were isolated from the pharynx (2.10%) and 30 from the nose (5.74%) (**Figure 3**). When analyzed by gender, 26 MRSA strains were isolated from males (63.41%) and 15 were isolated in females (36.59%). Besides, the age group 7–9 years was where more MRSA strains were found with 23 strains (4.39%, $p < 0.05$), followed by the age group 4–6 years with 8 (1.52%), 16–18 years with 5 strains (0.95%), 10–12 years with 4 strains (0.76%), while in children 1–3 only one MRSA strain was found (0.19%) and in the group 13–15, there was no isolation of MRSA strains (**Figure 1**).

Figure 4 shows the comparison of antibiotic resistance between MSSA and MRSA strains, the only antibiotic showing a significant difference was oxacillin ($p < 0.0001$). Similar to that shown in **Figure 2**, penicillin is the antibiotic to which both types of strains show the most resistance (93.17% and 84.21% between MRSA and MSSA strains respectively), followed by erythromycin (29.45% MRSA, 21.45% MSSA), clindamycin, ciprofloxacin, cephalothin, tetracycline, trimethoprim-sulfamethoxazole, macrolides (approximately 9% MRSA and 8% MSSA) and gentamicin (5.42% MRSA and 2.93% MSSA), no vancomycin-resistant strains were found.

3.3 MRSA strain typing

Table 3 shows the typing data of the 41 MRSA strains. It was found that 6 strains presented staphylococcal cassette chromosome (SCC*mec)* II (14.63%), 4 nasal (13.33%) and 2 pharyngeal (18.18%), so these would be HA-MRSA strains (14.64%). While 35 community-acquired MRSA strains were found (85.36%), of which 20

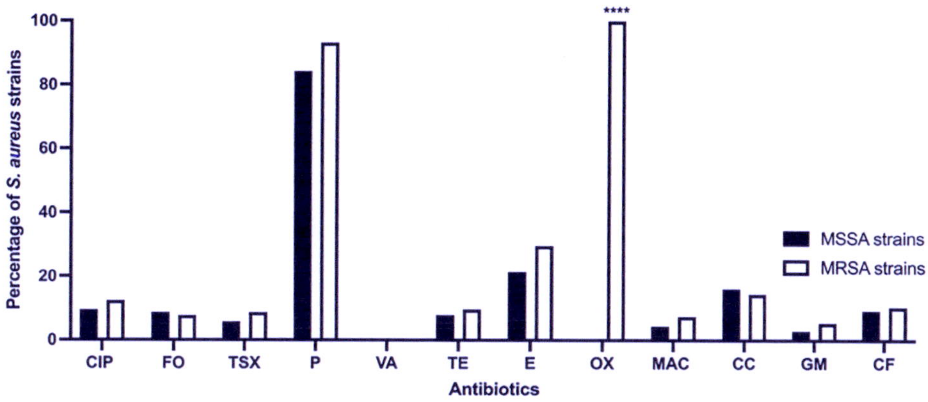

Figure 4.
Antibiotic resistance of MRSA and MSSA strains. CIP: ciprofloxacin, FO: fosfomycin. TSX: trimethoprim-sulfamethoxazole, P: penicillin, VA: vancomycin, TE: tetracycline, E: erythromycin, OX: oxacillin, MAC: macrolides, CC: clindamycin, GM: gentamicin, and CF: cephalothin. **** $p < 0.0001$.

Strain	Site	Gender	Age	*mecA*	*luk*-PV	*psm*	SCC*mec*	MRSA-type	*spa*-type
105 N	N	F	4	+	–	–	IV	CA-MRSA	t-527
106F	P	M	5	+	+	–	IV	CA-MRSA	t-527
120 N	N	M	5	+	–	–	IVa	CA-MRSA	t-6367
133F	P	M	6	+	+	–	IV	CA-MRSA	t-084
511 N	N	F	18	+	–	–	IV	CA-MRSA	t-8163
611 N	N	M	6	+	+	+	IV	CA-MRSA	t-909
612 N	N	M	6	+	–	–	IV	CA-MRSA	t-2651
617F	P	M	7	+	–	–	IV	CA-MRSA	t-14362
628 N	N	M	8	+	–	–	IVa	CA-MRSA	t-3380
635 N	N	M	7	+	–	+	IVa	CA-MRSA	t-16665
637 N	N	M	8	+	–	–	II	HA-MRSA	t-1406
638 N	N	M	8	+	–	–	IV	CA-MRSA	t-723
639 N	N	M	7	+	–	–	IVa	CA-MRSA	t-136
642 N	N	F	7	+	+	+	IV	CA-MRSA	t-723
644 N	N	F	7	+	–	–	IV	CA-MRSA	t-4976
645 N	N	M	8	+	–	+	IVa	CA-MRSA	t-645
647 N	N	F	7	+	–	–	IVa	CA-MRSA	t-922
657 N	N	F	8	+	–	–	IV	CA-MRSA	t-253
659 N	N	M	8	+	–	–	IV	CA-MRSA	t-4318
663F	P	F	8	+	–	–	II	HA-MRSA	t-909
667F	P	F	8	+	–	–	IV	CA-MRSA	t-253
677 N	N	F	9	+	–	–	IVa	CA-MRSA	t-1710
680 N	N	M	9	+	–	–	IV	CA-MRSA	t-701
687 N	N	M	10	+	–	+	IV	CA-MRSA	t-304

Strain	Site	Gender	Age	*mecA*	*luk*-PV	*psm*	SCC*mec*	MRSA-type	*spa*-type
689 N	N	M	8	+	–	–	IV	CA-MRSA	t-701
690 N	N	F	9	+	–	–	IV	CA-MRSA	t-4976
691 N	N	M	9	+	–	–	II	HA-MRSA	t-701
752 N	N	M	12	+	+	–	IVa	CA-MRSA	t-4468
754F	P	M	12	+	+	+	IVa	CA-MRSA	t-136
845 N	N	F	7	+	+	+	IV	CA-MRSA	t-189
980F	P	F	18	+	–	–	II	HA-MRSA	t-021
1236 N	N	M	6	+	–	+	II	HA-MRSA	t-346
1237 N	N	M	6	+	+	–	II	HA-MRSA	t-021
1251F	P	M	7	+	+	–	IV	CA-MRSA	t-5747
1293 N	N	M	17	+	+	–	V	CA-MRSA	t-209
1521F	P	F	18	+	–	–	IVa	CA-MRSA	t-02
1547F	P	F	17	+	–	–	IVa	CA-MRSA	t-3955
1631 N	N	M	10	+	–	–	IVa	CA-MRSA	t-012
1632 N	N	M	7	+	–	–	IVa	CA-MRSA	t-012
1638F	P	M	7	+	–	–	IVa	CA-MRSA	t-189
1705 N	N	F	2	+	–	+	IV	CA-MRSA	t-189

P: pharynx, N: nose, F: female, M: male, +: positive, –: negative, CA-MRSA: community methicillin-resistant S. aureus *strain, HA-MRSA: hospital methicillin-resistant* S. aureus *strain.*

Table 3.
Genotyping of MRSA strains isolated from pharynx and nose in children and adolescents.

strains were typed as SCC*mec* IV (48.78%), 15 were isolated from the nose (50%) and 5 from the pharynx (45.45%). The SCC*mec* IVa variant was found in 14 strains (34.14%), 10 nasal (33.33%) and 4 pharyngeal (36.36%), while SCC*mec* V was only found in one nasal strain.

All strains presented the *mecA* gene; in the case of the PVL gene, 10 strains presented it (24.39%), 4 pharyngeal strains and 6 nasal strains. For the phenol soluble modulin gene (*psm*) 9 strains were positive (21.95%), of which 8 corresponded to nasal strains and 1 to a pharyngeal strain (**Table 3**).

A great diversity of *spa*-types was found, the most repeated *spa*-type was t-189 in three strains, twice *spa*-types were found: t-012, t-136, t-253, t-527, t-701, t-723, t-909, t-1210 and t-4976, the other *spa*-types were only found in one strain each (**Table 3**).

4. Discussion

The importance of studying *S. aureus* carriers lies in the fact that these individuals are more likely to have a subsequent infection [3], and many apparently healthy children develop life-threatening infections as asymptomatic carriers of *S. aureus* [21]. Permanent colonization of MRSA strains can lead to an increase in infections by up to 25% [22]. This makes surveillance of children carrying or colonized by *S. aureus* an important prevention mechanism.

In this study, 62.55% of *S. aureus* carriers were found in the pediatric population studied; this value is higher than that found in other studies that found up to 40% of carriers [3]. We found that pharyngeal exclusive carriers were 21.47%, nasal exclusive carriers 13.74% and 27.31% in both sites carriers, highlighting that they are apparently healthy *S. aureus* carriers from daycare centers and schools, in this sense, Esposito et al.; in 2014 [23] investigated healthy school children and adolescents in Milan, Italy, reporting a 53% colonization by *S. aureus*, specifically 26% of pharyngeal carriers, 39% nasal and 12% in both sites, with results similar to those found in this work. However, colonization depends on the ecological niche; we found more pharyngeal than nasal carriers as reported in other studies [23–29].

Age plays an important role; it has been seen that children 12 months of age have a higher incidence of *S. aureus* bacteremia than older children. Low birth weight and earlier gestational age are considered risk factors for colonization and worse outcomes of *S. aureus* episodes [30].

In this sense, we found that colonization increases with age, with significance in the age groups 7–9 ($p < 0.05$) and 10–12 years ($p < 0.01$) with respect to the group of 1–3 years. This is in agreement with what was found in Spain where colonization increases above 5 years of age [3]. With respect to gender, significant differences were only found in nasal colonization, with women being more colonized than men ($p < 0.01$). There are reports of higher colonization in men, as well as living in urban areas, attending schools or daycare centers and presenting previous skin infections as well as chronic diseases (asthma, atopic dermatitis, allergies) [3].

Determining the type of methicillin resistance of *S. aureus* strains is important because MRSA and MSSA strains have different characteristics and pathogenicity [1, 5], this is also reflected in the clinic, as infections caused by MSSA strains are higher than those caused by MRSA strains [4], 72% of bacteremias and meningitis in infants are caused by MSSA strains [4]. In addition, MRSA and MSSA strains are the main responsible for skin and soft tissue infections in school-age children (6 to 11 years old in particular), being important that the same strain can cause repeated infections in up to 90% of the cases [31]. However, within the current epidemiology, MRSA has shown a downward trend with a decrease since the 2000s [4, 32], However, the opposite has been observed in MSSA strains, with an increase in their prevalence, which generates an increase in infections at hospital and community level. Therefore, MSSA infection has gained ground as there has been an increase in infections, which generates concern for a greater distribution of this strain at hospital and community level [4].

Regarding the type of *S. aureus* strains, we found a higher percentage of MSSA strains (92.16%) compared to MRSA strains (7.84%), these percentages are in agreement with the findings by Ericson et al. [4], which show that 72.1% of the infections are caused by MSSA against 27.9% produced by MRSA strains. However, our data are for colonization and not for infection, so the difference in the percentages may be because our study population is not hospitalized but community-based and apparently healthy.

MSSA strains were found in a higher percentage in the pharynx than the nose, unlike MRSA strains, which were found more in the nose than in the pharynx (**Figure 3**). In this regard, a study conducted in the USA found that *S. aureus* colonizes the nose between 28 and 32% [32], we only found 13.74% of carriers exclusively in the nose, but if we take into account carriers from both sites, the percentage is 35.21%, which is similar to the study by Macnow et al. [30]. However, the percentage of nasal

MRSA strains in that study ranged from 0.9% to 1.5%; we found a higher percentage of 5.74% nasal and 2.1% pharyngeal. This increase could be due to the difference in the country and the time of the study carried out, since there is a difference of more than ten years with respect to ours, and colonization by MRSA strains has been increasing as mentioned in other studies [5, 32, 33].

With respect to Mexico, studies regarding the colonization of *S. aureus* in the pediatric population are limited; it has been reported that in 2001 the prevalence of MRSA strains was 17 to 23%, but decreased to 4% in 2002, possibly due to control measures in hospitals [22]. In our study, we found a colonization of 7.04% of MRSA strain carriers in the community population studied, also different from the 1.44% reported in Spain [3], these differences are possibly due to the fact that these studies were carried out in hospitals, unlike ours, which is an apparently healthy community population.

In several studies carried out in various hospitals in Mexico, the presence of MRSA strains has been reported, mainly HA-MRSA strains, but the presence of CA-MRSA strains has also been reported, so that both types are circulating in hospitals [22]. In our study, we found more CA-MRSA strains (85.36%) than HA-MRSA (14.64%) which is expected since the population studied was not in hospitals. This also coincides with the fact that CA-MRSA strains have increased in the population [21, 32]. The infection rate in children by CA-MRSA strains varies according to the country. In Argentina, 65% of bacteremias in children are caused by CA-MRSA, in the USA 31.6% of infections by this strain were reported, while in Greece the CA-MRSA strain was identified in 35% of children with osteoarticular infection and 75% with pneumonia [3]. In our case, only 6% of people colonized with CA-MRSA strains were found, which is a low percentage compared to previous data, but it should be considered that the population studied is from the community and not hospitalized people.

Although the percentage of MRSA strains was low, this does not mean that the population studied is not at risk, since the percentage of MSSA strains was high and it has been shown that infant mortality after infection with MRSA or MSSA strains is similar [4]. However, MSSA strains cause more infections and deaths in infants than MRSA strains [4], therefore, infection prevention should include MSSA strains in addition to MRSA strains.

Another aspect to be reviewed is the antibiotic treatment of *S. aureus* infections in the pediatric population, which is a major challenge at present, so it is necessary to take into account the epidemiology, the type of exposure, the characteristics of the strain and the patient in order to provide adequate treatment [4, 11]. In this regard, MRSA and MSSA strains are susceptible to various antibiotics, and in this study, as in others, resistance to penicillin is very high [34, 35], In this study, we found around 90% of strains resistant to penicillin, erythromycin was the second most resistant antibiotic, the other antibiotics analyzed showed less than 20% resistance. In this regard, there are reports that MRSA strains are more resistant to antibiotics than MSSA strains [36–38], in our case was no exception and we found a difference of about 10% more MRSA strains than MSSA-resistant to penicillin and erythromycin, similar to other reports [3, 39, 40]. It should be noted that no vancomycin-resistant strains were found. When there is suspicion of infection by MRSA strains, the basis of treatment is usually vancomycin (vancomycin plus nafcillin or oxacillin), cephalosporins, clindamycin, linezolid or ceftaroline [9, 12]. Unfortunately, the literature mentions that there are pediatric populations that do not tolerate treatment with vancomycin, so alternatives such as daptomycin, ceftaroline and even linezolid should be chosen [9]. Another important aspect to consider is the timing of treatment. Currently, an adequate duration of antibiotic therapy in the pediatric population has not been established, so it is important to address this issue. There are proposals for temporality, which advise a duration of intravenous antibiotic therapy of 7–14 days and even up to 6 weeks in endocarditis [9]. Finally, antibiotic treatment depends on the type of *S. aureus* strain causing the infection and the characteristics of the host to avoid therapeutic failures and increased morbidity and mortality.

The infection generated by this bacterium is mediated by genetic factors, which determine its pathogenicity and virulence. All the MRSA strains isolated presented the *mecA* gene, 24.39% presented the PVL gene and 21.95% the *psm* gene, finding strains that presented both genes, which are CA-MRSA strains, it has been seen that these proteins are important for the pathology of the bacterium [41–44], strains carrying these genes are more virulent and should be under surveillance [43, 45, 46]. Finding these strains in the pediatric community is a call to be alert to their dissemination and to perform control measures.

The diversity of serotypes found in MRSA strains is very large, which speaks of the great variety of strains present in the community and the wide genetic variability of this bacterium, which has been previously reported [25, 47].

The host is another important factor in *S. aureus* infection and it has been seen that in children this bacterium can be found more commonly in sites other than the nose, such as the pharynx, inguinal folds, axillae, umbilicus and umbilicus [32, 48]. As was found in this study, there are more carriers in the pharynx than in the nose. Therefore, in high-risk populations, surveillance programs (nasal and pharyngeal screening) should be carried out to detect colonization by *S. aureus*. This has already been proven in decolonization protocols in orthopedic and cardiac surgery patients [4, 49]. Therefore, surveillance and decolonization programs in the pediatric population may help to decrease the rates of colonization, infection and death caused by *S. aureus*.

5. Conclusion

In this study, a high percentage of *S. aureus* carriers was found in the pediatric population studied. A greater number of *S. aureus* strains were isolated from the pharynx than from the nose. A higher presence of nasal *S. aureus* was found in women than in men ($p < 0.01$). Penicillin is the main antibiotic to which pharyngeal and nasal strains are resistant (>80%), followed by erythromycin (>30%), clindamycin and tetracycline (>15%). No strains resistant to vancomycin were found. The number of MSSA strains is higher than MRSA strains, a greater number of CA-MRSA than HA-MRSA strains were found, some with virulence factors such as PVL and *psm*. The *spa* types found were very diverse. Therefore, it is important to establish detection and decolonization programs in the pediatric population of the community to avoid possible infections and deaths caused by this bacterium.

Conflict of interest

The authors declare no conflict of interest.

Author details

Anaid Bustos-Hamdan[1], Samuel González García[2], Juan Antonio Guzmán Salgado[1], Aída Hamdan-Partida[1] and Jaime Bustos-Martínez[1*]

1 Departamento de Atención a la Salud, Universidad Autónoma Metropolitana – Xochimilco, Mexico City, Mexico

2 Doctorado en Ciencias Biológicas y de la Salud, Universidad Autónoma Metropolitana, Mexico City, Mexico

*Address all correspondence to: jbustos@correo.xoc.uam.mx

References

[1] Mlynarczyk-Bonikowska B, Kowalewski C, Krolak-Ulinska A, Marusza W. Molecular mechanisms of drug resistance in *Staphylococcus aureus*. International Journal of Molecular Sciences. 2022;**23**(15):8088

[2] Keim KC, Horswill AR. *Staphylococcus aureus*. Trends in Microbiology. 2023;**31**(12):1300-1301

[3] Del Rosal T, Méndez-Echevarría A, Garcia-Vera C, Escosa-Garcia L, Agud M, Chaves F, et al. *Staphylococcus aureus nasal* colonization in Spanish children. THE COSACO nationwide surveillance study. Infection and Drug Resistance. 2020;**13**:4643-4651

[4] Ericson JE, Popoola VO, Smith PB, Benjamin DK, Fowler VG, Benjamin DK, et al. Burden of invasive *Staphylococcus aureus* infections in hospitalized infants. JAMA Pediatrics. 2015;**169**(12):1105-1111

[5] Lee AS, de Lencastre H, Garau J, Kluytmans J, Malhotra-Kumar S, Peschel A, et al. Methicillin-resistant *Staphylococcus aureus*. Nature Reviews Disease Primers. 2018;**4**:18033

[6] Bustos-Martínez JA, Hamdan-Partida A, Gutiérrez-Cárdenas M. *Staphylococcus aureus*: The re-emergence of a pathogen in the community. Rev Bioméd. 2006;**17**(4):287-305

[7] Kalu IC, Kao CM, Fritz SA. Management and prevention of *Staphylococcus aureus* infections in children. Infectious Disease Clinics of North America. 2022;**36**(1):73-100

[8] González-García S, Hamdan-Partida A, Bustos-Hamdan A, Bustos-Martínez J. Factors of nasopharynx that favor the colonization and persistence of *Staphylococcus aureus*. In: Zhou X, Zhang Z, editors. Pharynx – Diagnosis and Treatment. London, UK, United Kingdom: IntechOpen; 2021. pp. 75-81

[9] McMullan BJ, Campbell AJ, Blyth CC, McNeil JC, Montgomery CP, Tong SYC, et al. Clinical management of *Staphylococcus aureus* bacteremia in neonates, children, and adolescents. Pediatrics. 2020;**146**(3):e20200134

[10] Campbell AJ, Al Yazidi LS, Phuong LK, Leung C, Best EJ, Webb RH, et al. Pediatric *Staphylococcus aureus* bacteremia: Clinical Spectrum and predictors of poor outcome. Clinical Infectious Diseases. 2022;**74**(4):604-613

[11] Newnam KM. Surveillance and isolation of methicillin-resistant *Staphylococcus aureus* colonization in the neonatal intensive care unit. Advances in Neonatal Care. 2016;**16**(4):298-307

[12] Oestergaard LB, Schmiegelow MDS, Bruun NE, Skov R, Andersen PS, Larsen AR, et al. *Staphylococcus aureus* bacteremia in children aged 5-18 years-risk factors in the new millennium. The Journal of Pediatrics. 2018;**203**:108-115.e3

[13] James G. Universal bacterial identification by PCR and DNA sequencing of 16S rRNA gene. In: Schuller M, Sloots T, James G, Halliday C, Carter I, editors. PCR for Clinical Microbiology. Dordrecht: Springer; 2010:209-214

[14] CLSI. Performance Standards for Antimicrobial Disk Suceptibility Test. 13th ed. Pennsylvania, Wayne: Clinical and Laboratory Standards Institute; 2018

[15] Oliveira DC, de Lencastre H. Multiplex PCR strategy for rapid

identification of structural types and variants of the mec element in methicillin-resistant *staphylococcus aureus*. Antimicrobial Agents and Chemotherapy. 2002;**46**(7):2155-2161

[16] Boye K, Bartels MD, Andersen IS, Møller JA, Westh H. A new multiplex PCR for easy screening of methicillin-resistant *Staphylococcus aureus* SCCmec types I–V. Clinical Microbiology and Infection. 2007;**13**(7):725-727

[17] Lina G, Piémont Y, Godail-Gamot F, Bes M, Peter MO, Gauduchon V, et al. Involvement of Panton-valentine leukocidin—Producing *Staphylococcus aureus* in primary skin infections and pneumonia. Clinical Infectious Diseases. 1999;**29**(5):1128-1132

[18] Mehlin C, Headley CM, Klebanoff SJ. An inflammatory polypeptide complex from *Staphylococcus epidermidis*: Isolation and characterization. The Journal of Experimental Medicine. 1999;**189**(6):907-918

[19] Shopsin B, Gomez M, Montgomery SO, Smith DH, Waddington M, Dodge DE, et al. Evaluation of protein a gene polymorphic region DNA sequencing for typing of *Staphylococcus aureus* strains. Journal of Clinical Microbiology. 1999;**37**(11):3556-3563

[20] Asghar AH. Molecular characterization of methicillin-resistant *Staphylococcus aureus* isolated from tertiary care hospitals. Pakistan Journal of Medical Sciences. 2014;**30**(4):698

[21] Immergluck LC, Leong T, Malhotra K, Parker TC, Ali F, Jerris RC, et al. Geographic surveillance of community associated MRSA infections in children using electronic health record data. BMC Infectious Diseases. 2019;**19**(1):170

[22] Ortíz-Gil MÁ, Cardona-Alvarado MI. The molecular epidemiological study of MRSA in Mexico. In: Bustos-Martínez J, Valdez-Alarcón JJ, editors. Staphylococcal Infections – Recent Advances and Perspectives. London, UK, United Kingdom: IntechOpen; 2023

[23] Esposito S, Terranova L, Zampiero A, Ierardi V, Rios WP, Pelucchi C, et al. Oropharyngeal and nasal *Staphylococcus aureus* carriage by healthy children. BMC Infectious Diseases. 2014;**14**:723

[24] Hamdan-Partida A, Sainz-Espuñes T, Bustos-Martínez J. Characterization and persistence of *Staphylococcus aureus* strains isolated from the anterior nares and throats of healthy carriers in a Mexican community. Journal of Clinical Microbiology. 2010;**48**(5):1701-1705

[25] Hamdan-Partida A, González-García S, de la Rosa GE, Bustos-Martínez J. Community-acquired methicillin-resistant *Staphylococcus aureus* can persist in the throat. International Journal of Medical Microbiology. 2018;**308**(4):469-475

[26] Nilsson P, Ripa T. *Staphylococcus aureus* throat colonization is more frequent than colonization in the anterior nares. Journal of Clinical Microbiology. 2006;**44**(9):3334-3339

[27] Mertz D, Frei R, Jaussi B, Tietz A, Stebler C, Flückiger U, et al. Throat swabs are necessary to reliably detect carriers of *Staphylococcus aureus*. Clinical Infectious Diseases. 2007;**45**(4):475-477

[28] Williamson DA, Ritchie S, Keren B, Harrington M, Thomas MG, Upton A, et al. Persistence, discordance and diversity of *Staphylococcus aureus* nasal and oropharyngeal colonization in school-aged children. The Pediatric Infectious Disease Journal. 2016;**35**(7):744-748

[29] González-García S, Hamdan-Partida A, Valdez-Alarcón JJ, Bustos-Hamdan A, Bustos-Martínez J. Main factors of *Staphylococcus aureus* associated with the interaction to the cells for their colonization and persistence. In: Bustos-Martínez J, Valdez-Alarcón JJ, editors. Staphylococcal Infections – Recent Advances and Perspectives. London, UK, United Kingdom: IntechOpen; 2023

[30] Mayorga Chavez D, Arnao Noboa A, Pereira OH. Risk factors associated with hospital stay in children with *Staphylococcus aureus* bacteremia. Revista Ecuatoriana de Pediatría. 2020;**21**(2):1-9

[31] Cane F, Posfay-Barbe KM, Pittet LF. Hygiene measures and decolonization of *Staphylococcus aureus* made simple for the pediatric practitioner. The Pediatric Infectious Disease Journal. 2024;**43**(5):e178-e182

[32] Macnow T, O'Toole D, DeLaMora P, Murray M, Rivera K, Whittier S, et al. Utility of surveillance cultures for antimicrobial resistant organisms in infants transferred to the neonatal intensive care unit. The Pediatric Infectious Disease Journal. 2013;**32**(12):e443-e450

[33] Rojo P, Barrios M, Palacios A, Gomez C, Chaves F. Community-associated *Staphylococcus aureus* infections in children. Expert Review of Anti-Infective Therapy. 2010;**8**(5):541-554

[34] Rao S, Linke L, Magnuson R, Jauch L, Hyatt DR. Antimicrobial resistance and genetic diversity of *Staphylococcus aureus* collected from livestock, poultry and humans. One Health. 2022;**11**(15):100407

[35] Vestergaard M, Frees D, Ingmer H. Antibiotic resistance and the MRSA problem. Microbiol Spectrum. 2019;**7**(2):10-1128. DOI: 10.1128/microbiolspec.gpp3-0057-2018

[36] Thompson T, Brown PD. Comparison of antibiotic resistance, virulence gene profiles, and pathogenicity of methicillin-resistant and methicillin-susceptible *Staphylococcus aureus* using a *Caenorhabditis elegans* infection model. Pathogens and Global Health. 2014;**108**(6):283

[37] Camacho-Cruz J, Gutiérrez IF, Brand-López K, Sosa-Rodríguez YA, Vásquez-Hoyos P, Gómez-Cortés LC, et al. Differences between methicillin-susceptible versus methicillin-resistant *Staphylococcus aureus* infections in pediatrics: Multicenter cohort study conducted in Bogotá, Colombia, 2014-2018. The Pediatric Infectious Disease Journal. 2022;**41**(1):12

[38] Rahimi F, Bouzari M, Katouli M, Pourshafie MR. Antibiotic resistance pattern of methicillin resistant and methicillin sensitive *Staphylococcus aur*eus isolates in Tehran, Iran. Jundishapur Journal of Microbiology. 2013;**6**(2):144-149

[39] Karabiber N, Dinc BM. Erythromycin-heteroresistant methicillin-resistant *Staphylococcus aureus* isolates from Turkey. Clinical Microbiology and Infection. 2008;**14**(6):626-627

[40] Zheng XY, Choy BNK, Zhou MM, Zhao ZY. Antibiotic resistance pattern of *Staphylococcus aureus* isolated from pediatrics with ocular infections: A 6-year hospital-based study in China. Frontiers in Pediatrics. 2021;**9**:728634

[41] Qu MD, Kausar H, Smith S, Lazar PG, Kroll-Desrosiers AR, Iii CH, et al. Epidemiological and clinical features of Panton-valentine Leukocidin positive *Staphylococcus aureus* bacteremia:

A case-control study. PLoS One. 2022;**17**(3):e0265476

[42] Vittorakis E, Vică ML, Zervaki CO, Vittorakis E, Maraki S, Mavromanolaki VE, et al. Examining the prevalence and antibiotic susceptibility of *S. Aureus* strains in hospitals: An analysis of the *pvl* gene and its Co-occurrence with other virulence factors. Microorganisms. 2023;**11**(4):841

[43] Bennett MR, Thomsen IP. Epidemiological and clinical evidence for the role of toxins in *S. Aureus* human disease. Toxins. 2020;**12**(6):408

[44] Lade H, Chung SH, Lee Y, Joo HS, Kim JS. Genotypes of Staphylococcus aureus clinical isolates are associated with phenol-soluble Modulin (PSM) production. Toxins. 2022;**14**(8):556

[45] Wu S, Zhang F, Huang J, Wu Q, Zhang J, Dai J, et al. Phenotypic and genotypic characterization of PVL-positive *Staphylococcus aureus* isolated from retail foods in China. International Journal of Food Microbiology. 2019;**304**:119-126

[46] Klein S, Hannesen J, Zanger P, Heeg K, Boutin S, Nurjadi D. Entry of Panton–valentine leukocidin-positive methicillin-resistant *Staphylococcus aureus* into the hospital: Prevalence and population structure in Heidelberg, Germany 2015-2018. Scientific Reports. 2020;**10**(1):13243

[47] Hamdan-Partida A, González-García S, Martínez-Ruíz FJ, Zavala-Sánchez MÁ, Bustos-Hamdan A, Bustos-Martínez J. Molecular characterization of *Staphylococcus aureus* strains isolated from mobile phones. Microorganisms. 2022;**10**(3):669

[48] Whittington KJ, Malone SM, Hogan PG, Ahmed F, Flowers J, Milburn G, et al. *Staphylococcus aureus* bacteremia in pediatric patients: Uncovering a rural health challenge. Open Forum Infectious Diseases. 2023;**10**(7):ofad296

[49] Chen AF, Wessel CB, Rao N. *Staphylococcus aureus* screening and decolonization in orthopaedic surgery and reduction of surgical site infections. Clinical Orthopaedics. 2013;**471**(7):2383-2399

Chapter 5

Current Insights and Future Directions in *Staphylococcus aureus* Infections: Advances and Perspectives

Sushama Agarwalla and Suhanya Duraiswamy

Abstract

Staphylococcus aureus infections are a global health concern, causing various illnesses. Recent research has provided insights into the epidemiology and pathogenesis of these infections, including the role of virulence factors and immune evasion strategies. Understanding the genetic mechanisms responsible for resistance is crucial in dealing with antibiotic-resistant strains like MRSA, which is the focus of this chapter. We also explore the advancements in diagnostics and detection methods, such as PCR and whole-genome sequencing and alternative treatments, *viz.* anti-virulence agents, monoclonal antibodies, and innovative antimicrobial peptides, which have improved patient outcomes. We end the chapter with a focus on the future research required for developing effective vaccines and alternative therapeutics to address the increasing concern of *Staphylococcus aureus* infections.

Keywords: *Staphylococcus aureus*, infections, epidemiology, pathogenesis, antibiotic resistance, diagnosis

1. Introduction

Staphylococcus aureus (*S. aureus*) is a Gram-positive bacterium that is part of the Staphylococcaceae family and is spherical in shape usually arranged in clusters [1, 2]. *S. aureus* has the ability to thrive in environments with varying levels of oxygen and has a diverse range of virulence factors that allow it to cause infections in humans posing a significant global health challenge [3]. *S. aureus* infections lead to various illness that span from minor skin and soft tissue inflammations, boils, and cellulitis to severe bloodstream infections—septicemia [4], endocarditis (infection of the heart valves), and pulmonary infections (pneumonia) [5]. They are responsible for *healthcare-associated infections* (HAIs) *or* nosocomial infections that occur in healthcare settings, commonly affecting individuals with compromised immune systems, or those with recent surgical procedures, or patients with invasive medical devices like catheters and/or ventilators [6] as well as *community-acquired infections* (CAI) manifesting as skin and wound infections, such as abscesses, as well as pneumonia in individuals

IntechOpen

who are otherwise healthy [7]. A strain of *S. aureus* that is resistant to numerous antibiotics, methicillin-resistant *S. aureus* (MRSA), poses significant challenges HAIs [8].

This study presents a broad overview of the latest findings and potential areas of exploration in the context of *S. aureus* infections, emphasizing recent progress and future possibilities. We first focus on the virulence, epidemiology, and pathogenesis of *S. aureus* infections [5]—recent research has provided valuable insights into the mechanisms used by *S. aureus* to cause persistent and recurrent infections, including the role of certain virulence factors and immune evasion strategies. We briefly look at these and move on to the progress made in diagnostics and detection methods—conventional methods for analyzing cultures can be quite time-consuming and may not always provide accurate results, resulting in delays in diagnosing conditions and potentially ineffective treatment. Nevertheless, advancements in molecular techniques, like polymerase chain reaction (PCR) and whole-genome sequencing, provide a swift and precise means of identifying *S. aureus* and its resistance profiles. These advancements hold promise in enhancing patient outcomes by enabling timely and precise antibiotic treatment.

We will then discuss the management and treatment of *S. aureus* infections. There have been growing concerns about the rising resistance to antibiotics, which has led to the investigation of alternative treatments *viz.* anti-virulence agents, monoclonal antibodies, and innovative antimicrobial peptides. Exploring alternative drug applications and advancing innovative treatment approaches, like phage therapy and immunotherapies, demonstrate potential in addressing *S. aureus* infections.

2. Regulation of *S. aureus* virulence factor

The regulation of virulence factors in *S. aureus* entails an intricate network that comprises interactions among genetic, biochemical, and environmental components. The regulatory mechanisms of *S. aureus* have a crucial function in its survival, pathogenicity, and adaptability and are essential for its capacity to attach to and infiltrate host tissues, avoid immune detection, and cause harm by means of toxins and enzymes. Understanding these virulence characteristics is important for the development of efficacious therapies and prevention measures against *S. aureus* infections.

The two-component system (TCS), a transcription regulator, plays a critical role in detecting environmental changes and converting them into coordinated regulatory reactions. Significantly, TCS systems, including the accessory gene regulator (*agr*) a quorum-sensing system and the *S. aureus* exoprotein expression (Sae) locus, are accountable for sensing and reacting to environmental stimuli. These pathways enable the regulation of toxins, surface proteins, and stress responses [9, 10]. In a typical TCS, an external signal activates a membrane-associated histidine kinase, leading to its autophosphorylation and subsequent phosphorylation of a response regulator. Once phosphorylated, the response regulator binds to specific DNA sequence motifs, thereby altering the expression of target genes. Most strains of *S. aureus* encode 16 different TCSs [11, 12], with one being essential (WalKR), while the other 15 can be inactivated [13, 14]. Notably, TCSs such as AgrAC, SaeRS, and ArlRS are directly linked to *S. aureus* virulence and regulate a large number of host-impacting secreted proteins.

The *agr* system, first described in 1986, is the most extensively studied and functions as a master virulence regulator through a quorum-sensing mechanism [9] to detect population density and regulate the expression of virulence factors accordingly.

Regulatory system	Components	Key functions and features
Two-Component Systems	AgrAC, SaeRS, ArlRS	• Detect environmental signals • Regulate expression of host-impacting proteins [15].
Accessory Gene Regulator (*agr*)	*agrA*, *agrC*, *agrD*, *agrB*	• Quorum-sensing system • Master regulator of virulence genes [9, 16–23].
Essential TCS	WalKR	• Essential for cell viability • Regulates cell wall metabolism and division [24].
SarA Protein Family	SarA, Rot, MgrA	• Transcriptional regulators • Modulate expression of a wide range of virulence genes [25–28].
Alternative Sigma Factors	SigB, SigH	• Regulate stress response and virulence gene expression under different environmental conditions [29, 30].

Table 1.
Summary of key regulatory systems in S. aureus.

The SaeRS and ArlRS systems are involved in responding to specific environmental stimuli, such as changes in temperature, pH, and the presence of antimicrobial agents, thus modulating the expression of genes necessary for survival and pathogenicity. In addition to TCSs, *S. aureus* employs several cytoplasmic regulators like the SarA protein family of transcriptional regulators to adapt and survive in the host environment by modulating the expression of virulence genes in response to environmental and intracellular signals [11]. **Table 1** summarizes the critical features and interplay of each system, elucidating their roles in the regulation of *S. aureus* virulence.

Although there are multiple regulators in the area, this chapter will not delve into discussing them. However, readers who are interested may refer to a comprehensive review [15] and other literatures for more detailed information [15, 31–35].

3. Epidemiology of *S. aureus* infections

The incidence and spread of *S. aureus* infections (both HAIs and CAIs) exhibit variabilities among several geographical areas and populations [5, 36]. MRSA is the cause of about 20–30% of *S. aureus* cases in HAIs [37]. They are linked to higher fatality rates in comparison to infections caused by methicillin-susceptible *S. aureus* (MSSA).

Some common risk factors for *S. aureus HAI* are:

a. *Hospitalization*: The act of being admitted to a hospital raises the likelihood of contracting *S. aureus* infections [38], which includes both MSSA and MRSA [39].

b. *Invasive devices,* such as central venous catheters, urinary catheters, and surgical implants, can serve as entrance routes for *S. aureus* to cause infections [40].

c. *Surgical site infections caused by S. aureus:* Surgical site infections (SSIs) resulting from *S. aureus* are a frequent and important complication that occurs after surgical procedures [41]. *S. aureus* is a bacteria that is often found on the skin and in the nasal passages, pharynx [42], and other areas of the body in individuals who are in good health. Nevertheless, it has the potential to induce infections once entering the body *via* surgical incisions or wounds causing both superficial and deep SSIs [43]. SSIs affect the skin and subcutaneous tissue, whereas deep SSIs affect tissues or organs that are located further under the surface. SSIs can manifest as erythema, edema, discomfort, and exudate at the surgical site [44]. Multiple variables contribute to the occurrence of *S. aureus* infections in surgical sites. Failure to adhere to appropriate infection control protocols, such as maintaining a sterile environment and using clean devices, heightens the likelihood of *S. aureus* contamination. Initially, the bacteria carries a multitude of virulence characteristics (sticky proteins, poisons, and enzymes) that enable it to attach to and infiltrate tissues, evade the immune response, and induce tissue harm [45].

d. *Specific patient characteristics/Vulnerable populations:* People who have certain underlying medical conditions as well as the elderly may be more vulnerable to *S. aureus* infections due to immune system dysfunction [46, 47]. For example:

- Preexisting medical disorders, such as diabetes or obesity, can heighten the vulnerability to *S. aureus* infections.

- Human Immunodeficiency Virus/Acquired Immunodeficiency Syndrome (HIV/AIDS) compromises immune function and raises susceptibility to several infections [48], including *S. aureus*.

- Patients with cancer who are receiving chemotherapy or radiation therapy also have compromised immune systems [48], which increases their susceptibility to *S. aureus* infections [49].

- Patients in intensive care units (ICUs), who may be exposed to elevated amounts of antibiotics and have weakened immune systems, are more susceptible to developing *S. aureus* infections [50].

- Patients with chronic lung disorders like Chronic Obstructive Pulmonary Disease (COPD) or asthma are prone to *S. aureus* lung infections due to their compromises lung function [51] and weak immune system.

- The immune system can be weakened by advanced kidney illness, making one more vulnerable to *S. aureus* infections, especially bloodstream infections [52].

- Individuals with autoimmune illnesses [53] are more susceptible to *S. aureus* infections due to immune system malfunction.

- Individuals who get organ transplants frequently use immunosuppressive drugs, which impair immune function and raise the risk of *S. aureus* infections [54].

- Immune system deterioration resulting from underlying cardiac problems [5] may heighten the vulnerability to bloodstream infections caused by *S. aureus*.

These are but a few instances of the many additional variables that can compromise immunity and raise the possibility of *S. aureus* infections.

S. aureus infections can impact people of all age groups in the community [55], without the need for prior contact with healthcare facilities. Community-acquired MRSA (CA-MRSA) infections are influenced by certain risk factors, which include:

a. *Skin integrity*: Skin infections, such as lacerations, punctures, or abrasions, serve as portals of entry for *S. aureus* to initiate infections [5].

b. *Close contact: S. aureus* is transmitted *via* direct skin-to-skin contact or contact with infected surfaces, making densely populated venues like schools, daycares, and athletic facilities possible sources of transmission. Athletes engaged in contact sports and activities, such as wrestling or football, face an elevated risk of contracting *S. aureus* skin infections, commonly referred to as "athlete's skin."

c. *Sharing:* Injection drug use can result in *S. aureus* bloodstream infections when individuals share infected needles and drug equipment [56].

d. *Insufficient hygiene*: Inadequate adherence to hand hygiene practices and lack of cleanliness can facilitate the spread of *S. aureus* in the population [57].

It should be emphasized that although particular populations may have a greater susceptibility to *S. aureus* infections, anybody has the potential to contract an infection. Implementing effective preventative measures, such as maintaining proper personal hygiene, consistently practicing handwashing, and adhering to appropriate infection control protocols, is essential for minimizing the spread and morbidity of *S. aureus* infections.

4. Clinical manifestations and treatment of *S. aureus* infections

From a clinical perspective, infections caused by *S. aureus* can exhibit a range of variations. The diagnosis and treatment of these infections are contingent upon the specific kind of infection and the features of the patient. *This information does not serve as a replacement for expert medical counsel, and it is crucial to seek guidance from a healthcare professional for individualized evaluation and treatment. S. aureus* infections can be categorized into bloodstream/cardiac, skin/soft tissue, respiratory, and bone/joint infections.

4.1 Bacteremia

Bacteremia is a critical medical condition characterized by the presence of bacteria in the bloodstream. It can occur due to initial infections [55], invasive medical procedures, or infections associated with implanted medical devices. Severe complications may occur, potentially resulting in sepsis, a serious systemic infection [56] that can be life-threatening. Understanding the clinical presentation of bacteremia [57] is crucial in order to quickly identify and treat the responsible organism, as different infections can have varying symptoms.

Antibiotics that are directed at the pathogen are the most important part of treatment. They stop bacteremia from getting worse and lower the risk of problems. Extensive study in academic contexts is necessary to advance our understanding of bacteremia.

4.1.1 Endocarditis

Endocarditis resulting from the damage to the inner lining and valves of the heart, often occurs after bacteremia. Common symptoms of this condition may include fever, a cardiac murmur, fatigue, night sweats, and difficulty breathing. Diagnosis requires blood cultures and echocardiograms, while treatment generally involves the administration of long-term intravenous antibiotics. There are instances where surgical intervention becomes necessary to repair or replace heart valves that have been affected.

4.2 Cutaneous and subcutaneous infections

S. aureus is capable of causing a range of infections affecting the skin and underlying soft tissues, such as furuncles, clusters of furuncles, localized collections of pus, inflammation of the skin and subcutaneous tissues [58], and infections in wounds. The clinical manifestations encompass erythema, edema, discomfort, and increased temperature at the site of infection. The diagnosis is typically made by evaluating the patient's clinical symptoms; however, in severe cases or when the infection does not improve with initial therapy, cultures and laboratory tests may be performed. The treatment typically includes the surgical opening and removal of abscesses, as well as the administration of antibiotics [59], which is determined by the seriousness and site of the infection [60].

4.2.1 Abscesses and boils

Abscesses and boils are localized formations of pus caused by infection. They appear as painful, swollen masses filled with pus, often accompanied by redness and swelling in the surrounding area. Diagnosis of these conditions is achieved through a clinical examination and the analysis of pus samples. Treatment involves the drainage of abscesses and the administration of antibiotics [61].

4.2.2 Cellulitis

Cellulitis is a bacterial illness that affects the skin and tissues underneath [62]. It causes the skin to become red, swollen, heated, and painful. Diagnosis is achieved by means of clinical examination and occasionally validated with blood tests or cultures obtained from the afflicted region. Treatment entails the administration of antibiotics either by the mouth or through a vein, depending on the seriousness of the condition [63].

4.2.3 Impetigo

Impetigo, a highly transmissible dermatological infection prevalent among youngsters, results in the formation of red sores or blisters that burst, discharge fluid, and develop a yellow-brown scab. The diagnosis is established by doing a clinical examination and culturing the lesion. Treatment options include the use of topical or oral antibiotics.

4.3 Infections of the bones and joints

4.3.1 Osteomyelitis

Osteomyelitis, a bone infection, manifests as localized discomfort, elevated body temperature, inflammation, and increased heat [64]. The diagnosis is established by doing blood tests, imaging examinations such as X-rays or MRIs, and performing a bone sample. The treatment for this condition typically entails the administration of extended courses of antibiotics, and in certain cases, surgical intervention may be necessary to excise the contaminated bone.

4.3.2 Septic arthritis

Septic arthritis, a condition characterized by infection within a joint leading to inflammation, manifests as intense joint pain, edema, redness, and fever [65]. Diagnosis of the condition is achieved by analyzing joint fluid and conducting blood tests. Treatment involves administering antibiotics and draining the infected joint fluid [66].

4.4 Pneumonia

S. aureus pneumonia [67] can occur as either a primary infection or a secondary infection subsequent to influenza or other respiratory illnesses. Common symptoms of this condition may encompass coughing, chest discomfort, elevated body temperature, respiratory distress, and a productive cough accompanied by thick, pus-filled mucus. The diagnosis is usually made by conducting a comprehensive clinical assessment, along with performing chest imaging (such as chest X-ray), analyzing sputum cultures, and examining blood cultures. The treatment for *S. aureus* pneumonia typically involves the administration of intravenous antibiotics that are effective against the infections [68].

4.5 Management and treatment of infections caused by S. aureus

4.5.1 Preventive measures

Preventive measures are essential in reducing the occurrence and transmission of *S. aureus* infections [5]. Strict adherence to infection control protocols is crucial in preventing HAIs. Thorough hand hygiene practices are essential, including washing hands with soap and water or using alcohol-based hand sanitizers. It is important for healthcare providers to wear the necessary personal protective equipment, including gloves, gowns, and masks, when required.

Screening individuals by using either nasopharyngeal and pharyngeal swabs who may be at risk for *S. aureus* infections, such as those with a history of previous infections or colonization, can be an effective way to identify carriers of the bacteria, in addition to implementing infection control measures. Separating individuals who test positive for MRSA can effectively halt the transmission of the bacteria to other patients.

4.5.2 Antibiotics

When it comes to treating *S. aureus* infections, the selection of antibiotics is customized based on the strain's susceptibility and the severity of the illness. Typically, beta-lactam antibiotics such as penicillin or cephalosporins are effective against methicillin-sensitive strains. Alternatively, methicillin-resistant strains necessitate the use of different antibiotics like vancomycin, daptomycin, or linezolid. By conducting susceptibility testing, one can ascertain the most suitable antibiotic for specific cases.

4.5.3 Surgical intervention

In more serious instances or when the infection is not showing improvement with antibiotic treatment alone, surgical intervention may be required. One aspect of this work may include the removal of abscesses or infected implants to eradicate the infection and facilitate the healing process.

4.5.4 Vaccines

Continual research is also dedicated to the development of vaccines against *S. aureus* to proactively prevent infections. However, it is important to note that there is not yet an approved vaccine against *S. aureus*.

5. Antibiotic resistance in *S. aureus*

Antibiotics are frequently the only option for treating serious bacterial infections, particularly when alternative treatments have been unsuccessful or when the infection presents a substantial health hazard. Their capacity to specifically target and eradicate bacteria has rendered them indispensable in contemporary medicine [69]. Antibiotics are specifically engineered to target particular bacteria or impede their proliferation and can be categorized into the following [70]:

- Penicillins, amoxicillin, and ampicillin, which are commonly prescribed for respiratory, skin, and urinary tract infections [71];

- Cephalosporins, such as cephalexin and ceftriaxone, which have a broader spectrum of activity and are used for more severe infections or when resistance to penicillins is suspected;

- Macrolides, such as erythromycin, clarithromycin, and azithromycin, which are typically used for respiratory tract infections and some sexually transmitted diseases;

- Fluoroquinolones, such as ciprofloxacin and levofloxacin, which are effective against a wide range of infections, including urinary tract infections, respiratory infections, and certain gastrointestinal infections.

- Vancomycin and Linezolid are frequently prescribed medicines for the treatment of MRSA and are effective against numerous Gram-positive bacteria.

Antibiograms and minimum inhibitory concentration (MIC) testing are critical tools in combating antibiotic resistance in *S. aureus*. These tests allow healthcare professionals to determine the susceptibility or resistance of bacterial strains to specific antibiotics. Regularly conducting antibiograms helps healthcare facilities monitor resistance patterns and make informed decisions about appropriate antibiotic treatment. Determining MIC of oxacillin is essential in identifying MRSA strains. A higher MIC of oxacillin compared to methicillin-susceptible strains indicates the presence of MRSA. By utilizing antibiograms and MIC testing, healthcare providers can accurately diagnose MRSA infections and tailor treatment accordingly. This is crucial for effective treatment, preventing the spread of MRSA, and improving patient outcomes.

In clinical practice, the administration of certain antibiotics is usually determined by considering the type and severity of the infection, as well as the susceptibility of the bacteria [72]. In cases of severe bacterial infections, such as sepsis, initial treatment may involve the use of *broad-spectrum antibiotics* like cephalosporins or fluoroquinolones [73]. This is done to offer immediate coverage until specific culture findings are obtained.

Although antibiotics have a crucial role, their usage is filled with difficulties mainly due to the over prescription and improper use of antibiotics, which greatly contribute to the emergence of antibiotic or antimicrobial resistance (AMR). AMR arises when bacteria are exposed to antibiotics multiple times and evolve methods by spontaneous genetic mutations or horizontal gene transfer from other bacteria to avoid their effects, making the medications less potent [74] as well as leading to the survival and multiplication of resistant bacteria. The phenomenon of resistance can disseminate worldwide, thereby rendering the treatment of illnesses that were previously susceptible to antibiotics progressively more challenging.

AMR in *S. aureus*, including strains like MRSA and Vancomycin-resistant *S. aureus* (VRSA), mostly occurs due to the acquisition of resistance genes found on mobile genetic components like plasmids or through changes in the chromosomes (for example, the *mecA* gene found in MRSA) that modify the locations targeted by antibiotics [75]. The *mecA* gene produces penicillin-binding protein 2a (PBP2a), which decreases the effectiveness of beta-lactam antibiotics such as methicillin and penicillin by enabling the bacteria to persist in synthesizing their cell walls [76]. However, VRSA develops resistance by acquiring the vanA gene cluster, which is usually obtained through the transfer of genes from vancomycin-resistant *Enterococcus via* horizontal gene transfer. The vanA gene modifies the peptidoglycan structure of the bacterial cell wall, hence diminishing the binding affinity and efficacy of vancomycin, which is a crucial antibiotic used as a last option [77].

In addition, strains of *S. aureus* have the ability to deactivate beta-lactam antibiotics by producing beta-lactamases through *enzymatic processes* [78]. Increased production of efflux pumps, which are specialized transporter proteins used by bacteria to expel antibiotics from their cellular interior to the external environment, reduces the intracellular concentration of the drug and contributes to antibiotic resistance. In addition, *S. aureus biofilms*, which are complex bacterial communities enclosed by an extracellular matrix, serve as a protective barrier against antibiotics. This barrier prevents the effective penetration of drugs and provides a safe-haven for persister cells that have an increased tolerance to antibiotics.

The complex mechanisms involved highlight the challenges posed by antibiotic-resistant *S. aureus* infections, where in certain instances, combination therapy with multiple antibiotics may be necessary to effectively treat infections that are resistant to standard treatment. This also underscores the urgent requirement for inventive strategies to address AMR in clinical environments as well as requiring ongoing research into creative treatment techniques and strong surveillance measures to effectively address these changing threats [79]. With the aim of tackling the emergence of AMR, *antimicrobial stewardship programs* promote the prudent utilization of antibiotics. This involves ensuring that prescriptions are appropriate, with the correct dosage and duration of treatment, to minimize the likelihood of resistance. In addition, healthcare practitioners stress the significance of responsible antibiotic utilization, which encompasses the practice of prescription antibiotics only when they are medically required, ensuring that patients adhere to the entire prescribed antibiotic regimen and refraining from using antibiotics for viral illnesses. Furthermore, continuous investigation into novel medicines and alternative therapies is important to tackle the escalating menace of AMR.

To summarize, antibiotics are typically used as a final option for treating serious bacterial illnesses, with different varieties designed to specifically target pathogen. It is imperative to implement stringent infection control measures, adopt proper Ab prescribing practices, and advance the discovery of novel antibiotics and alternative treatment techniques to effectively combat the proliferation of AMR *S. aureus*, which poses a significant risk to public health. All these also highlight the importance of proper diagnostic strategies that are readily available at the healthcare settings for proper prescriptions, which is discussed in the following section.

6. Diagnosis and detection of *S. aureus* infections

The diagnosis of *S. aureus* infections is a critical aspect of clinical microbiology [80]; although there may be instances of mild cases, infections caused by *S. aureus* have the potential to become serious and even result in death if not accurately diagnosed and appropriately treated. Prompt medical intervention is essential to avert any negative consequences. The diagnosis of infection encompasses various laboratory techniques including culture-based methods [81], molecular technique such as PCR [82], and serological assays [83]. Each method has its own set of advantages and challenges, and recent advances have enhanced their accuracy and efficiency. This section provides a detailed overview of these diagnostic approaches, emphasizing their significance and application in the detection of *S. aureus* infections.

6.1 Culture-based techniques: gold standards

The diagnosis of *S. aureus* infections still relies on culture-based approaches, which include carefully isolating and identifying the bacteria from clinical samples [84]. This is done by allowing the organism to grow on selected media under controlled conditions. The method begins by collecting various clinical samples, such as blood, pus, or nasal swabs, which are then placed onto specialized media, such as blood agar or mannitol salt agar. After being inoculated, the plates are carefully placed in an incubator and kept at temperatures usually between 35 and 37°C for a duration of 18–24 hours.

The identification of *S. aureus* colonies relies mostly on their unique morphological traits, the observed hemolysis patterns on blood agar, and the distinctive color changes displayed by colonies on the medium. Confirming the identity of *S. aureus* requires the coagulase and catalase tests: coagulase test is essential for distinguishing between coagulase-positive *S. aureus* [85] and coagulase-negative staphylococci [86]. This distinction is significant for making clinical decisions since coagulase-positive strains are associated with virulence factors. Catalase testing is useful for differentiating between staphylococci, which produce catalase, and *streptococci*, which do not produce catalase. This helps in accurately identifying the species.

6.1.1 Advantages and challenges

Although culture-based techniques are widely regarded as the most reliable method for identifying and assessing the susceptibility of bacteria, they present notable difficulties. These tests are very time-consuming, usually taking up to 48 hours to receive definitive results, which can cause a delay in starting targeted medication. Moreover, these approaches require laboratory professionals who are highly skilled in microbiological methods to accurately carry out and analyze the tests. Ultimately, culture-based methods continue to be essential in clinical microbiology due to their reliability and ability to provide a thorough profile of bacteria [87].

6.2 Serological assays

Serological assays play a crucial role in diagnosing systemic *S. aureus* infections and establishing past exposure by detecting particular antibodies or antigens linked to the pathogen [83]. Enzyme immunoassays (EIAs) and latex agglutination tests are commonly used among these assays. EIAs detect the presence of antigens, such as protein A or clumping factor, by using antibodies tagged with enzymes. These antibodies can identify antigen-antibody complexes, providing a clear indication of the presence of *S. aureus*. The process entails applying antibodies onto a surface, introducing the sample, and utilizing enzyme-labeled antibodies to attach to any existing antigen-antibody complexes [88]. This leads to a detectable signal, usually in the form of a color alteration. In contrast, latex agglutination assays identify surface proteins such as coagulase and protein A by utilizing latex particles that are covered with antibodies. These antibodies clump together, or agglutinate, when they come into contact with certain antigens, thus indicating the presence of *S. aureus* visibly [89].

6.2.1 Advantages and challenges

These assays are highly regarded for their noninvasive characteristics, as they use serum or plasma samples and provide rapid responses within minutes to hours. Although they have benefits, problems like the possibility of reacting with comparable antigens from other organisms and the restricted ability to measure quantities, mostly in a qualitative or semiquantitative manner, emphasize the importance of cautious interpretation in clinical contexts. However, serological assays continue to be crucial for quick and noninvasive detection of *S. aureus*, aiding in prompt clinical decision-making.

6.3 Molecular techniques

Molecular techniques, particularly PCR, have revolutionized the diagnosis of *S. aureus* infections by enabling rapid and precise identification of the bacterium's genetic material [90].

6.3.1 Conventional PCR

It targets specific genes essential for *S. aureus* identification, such as nuc (encoding thermonuclease) and *mecA* (associated with methicillin resistance) [91, 92]. The process involves isolating DNA from clinical samples, amplifying target sequences using specific primers that flank the target gene regions, and visualizing the resulting amplified products through gel electrophoresis. This method allows for the detection and confirmation of *S. aureus* presence based on the presence or absence of specific DNA bands of expected sizes.

6.3.2 Real-time PCR (qPCR) for quantitative analysis

It enhances this process by enabling quantification of DNA in real-time during amplification [93]. It employs fluorescent dyes or probes that bind specifically to the amplified DNA, allowing for continuous monitoring of DNA accumulation as the reaction progresses. Real-time PCR [94] offers several advantages over conventional PCR, including faster turnaround times, as results can be obtained within hours rather than days, and the ability to provide quantitative data, which is crucial for determining the amount of target DNA present.

With multiplex PCR techniques, it becomes possible to detect multiple pathogens and resistance genes [90] all at once in a single assay.

6.3.3 Loop-mediated isothermal amplification (LAMP) for rapid diagnostics

Loop-mediated isothermal amplification (LAMP) is another molecular technique gaining prominence for its simplicity and rapidity [95]. LAMP amplifies DNA under isothermal conditions, meaning it operates at a constant temperature, typically between 60 and 65°C, using a set of four to six primers that recognize multiple regions within the target gene. This method does not require thermal cycling, which simplifies the process and reduces the equipment needed, making it suitable for resource-limited settings or point-of-care diagnostics [96].

6.3.4 Advantages and challenges

Molecular techniques play a crucial role in the rapid and accurate diagnosis of *S. aureus* infections, guiding appropriate treatment decisions and infection control measures. Continuous advancements in technology and methodologies promise to further enhance the sensitivity, specificity, and accessibility of these diagnostic tools, ultimately improving patient outcomes and public health responses to *S. aureus* infections and antibiotic resistance. Despite their advantages, molecular techniques also pose challenges. The initial setup costs for equipment such as thermal cyclers and real-time PCR machines, as well as the ongoing expense of reagents and consumables, can be prohibitive for some laboratories. Furthermore, the complexity of interpreting results and the requirement for trained personnel proficient in molecular biology techniques necessitate ongoing investment in training and quality assurance.

6.4 Advances and challenges in lab diagnosis of *S. aureus* infections

The diagnosis of *S. aureus* infections employs a range of laboratory techniques, each with distinct advantages and challenges. Culture-based methods remain the gold standard, while molecular techniques offer rapid and precise detection. Serological assays provide valuable insights into systemic infections. Advances in diagnostic technologies continue to enhance the accuracy and efficiency of *S. aureus* detection, but challenges such as antibiotic resistance and cost remain significant. Understanding and optimizing these diagnostic approaches are crucial for effective clinical management of *S. aureus* infections.

Recent developments using automated systems have significantly enhanced efficiency and speed revolutionizing both culture-based and molecular methods, significantly minimizing errors and delivering swift results [97]. Performing diagnostic tests at the patient's bedside provides rapid results [98]. Nevertheless, the absence of standardized protocols for certain assays presents a significant challenge, as it results in variability in outcomes and hampers the ability to interpret and compare data across different laboratories. Addressing these challenges is essential to ensure precise and prompt diagnostics for every patient.

7. Future perspectives and research directions

Successful treatment and preventative strategies depend on understanding the virulence, epidemiology, and pathophysiology of *S. aureus* infections. The survival and pathogenicity of *S. aureus* are significantly influenced by the control of its virulence components, such as the two-component system and cytoplasmic regulators. Targeted therapy development can be facilitated by an understanding of regulatory processes. Technological developments in diagnostics and detection, such molecular approaches, have the potential to improve patient outcomes by facilitating accurate and timely administration of antibiotics. Furthermore, the growing resistance to antibiotics emphasizes the need for substitute therapies including monoclonal antibodies, antivirulence medicines, and creative antimicrobial peptides. *S. aureus* infections necessitate a customized assessment and course of care, specifically for serious illnesses like bacteremia and endocarditis; additional research is required to increase diagnostic precision and create more potent treatment plans.

7.1 Conventional research for vaccines development

Conventionally research in tackling infections has been focused on the study and development of vaccines and antimicrobial medicines. Researchers work to find safe and efficient ways to fight different infections through comprehensive laboratory testing, clinical trials, and focused studies. The development of a potent vaccination against *S. aureus* is a viable strategy. The primary objective is to find antigens that can elicit effective immune responses and develop vaccine formulations that specifically target strains or virulence characteristics. Multiple vaccine candidates are presently undergoing preclinical or clinical studies.

7.2 Challenges and possibilities in preventing and controlling *S. aureus* infections amidst the rise of antibiotic resistance

AMR, or the emergence and spread of strains resistant to antibiotics, might compromise the efficacy of vaccinations and cause diseases that were previously eradicated. AMR diminishes the effectiveness of antibiotics in treating illnesses, potentially leading to extended illness, elevated healthcare expenses, and elevated death rates. AMR may potentially reverse the progress gained in the fight against disease eradication when it comes to vaccinations by making some bacterial diseases more challenging to treat and manage. This has necessitated the need for alternative antimicrobial drugs to provide alternative treatment choices. Research is being conducted to investigate innovative antimicrobial agents, including antimicrobial peptides, bacteriophages, and immune-based therapeutics. These techniques focus on distinct mechanisms of action, which could potentially make them effective against strains of drugs that have developed resistance. Anti-virulence techniques focus on impeding the development or function of virulence factors, which play a critical role in the pathogenicity of *S. aureus*, instead of directly killing the bacteria. By diminishing the bacteria's capacity to induce illness, these approaches can potentially mitigate the intensity of infections and augment the efficacy of current medications.

Enhancements in surveillance systems and diagnostic tests play a crucial role in identifying and monitoring the appearance and transmission of multidrug-resistant *S. aureus* strains and for devising specific treatment approaches. Gaining insight into the mechanisms that contribute to the transmission and dissemination of *S. aureus* in community settings is crucial for successful prevention and control. Antimicrobial stewardship involves ongoing initiatives to encourage the responsible use of antibiotics, which includes prescribing them appropriately and using de-escalation procedures. Implementing additional measures for infection control, such as rigorous cleaning standards, increased compliance with hand hygiene practices, and the application of antimicrobial coatings on surfaces, can effectively decrease the spread and acquisition of *S. aureus* infections. The advancement and assessment of novel treatment methods, such as the use of multiple therapies, approaches that target biofilms, present promising ways to combat antibiotic resistance in *S. aureus.*

7.3 Current developments in the study and treatment of *S. aureus* infections

The influence of host factors, such as weakened immune systems, coexisting medical conditions, and genetic predispositions, on the vulnerability to and consequences of *S. aureus* infections is currently being actively studied. Gaining insight into the interactions between hosts and pathogens can provide valuable guidance for tailoring individualized treatment strategies and prevention measures. Advancements are being made in the development of more efficient and precise procedures for assessing the susceptibility of microorganisms to antimicrobial agents. These methods will assist in choosing suitable medicines and provide guidance for personalized treatment approaches for *S. aureus* infections.

7.4 Developments in diagnostics of *S. aureus* infections

Swift diagnostic methods capable of detecting antibiotic resistance genes and forecasting antimicrobial susceptibility will facilitate prompt, focused, effective treatment, and management, ultimately contributing to the prevention and control of these infections. Traditional methods, such as culture and identification from clinical samples, can be time-consuming and require skilled laboratory personnel. Rapid diagnostic methods like PCR assays and Nucleic acid amplification techniques (NAATs) have been developed to detect *S. aureus* DNA within hours, enabling quicker diagnosis and appropriate therapy. Point-of-care tests are being developed to provide rapid results, reducing transmission risk in community settings.

8. Conclusions

As concluding remarks, we would like to summarize those future directions in combating *S. aureus* infections, particularly amidst escalating antibiotic resistance, involving multifaceted strategies aimed at enhancing treatment and control measures. Primary efforts include advancing vaccine development targeting specific antigens to stimulate robust immune responses and potentially reduce transmission rates. Simultaneously, research into alternative antimicrobial agents like antimicrobial peptides, bacteriophages, and immune-based therapies seeks to broaden therapeutic options against resistant strains. Antivirulence strategies, which focus on neutralizing virulence factors rather than solely eradicating bacteria, show promise in mitigating infection severity and optimizing current treatment efficacy. Addressing challenges involves bolstering surveillance systems to monitor multidrug-resistant strains, advancing rapid diagnostic technologies for predicting antibiotic resistance, and promoting antimicrobial stewardship to foster responsible antibiotic use and combat resistance emergence. Implementation of stringent infection control measures and continued exploration of innovative treatment modalities are essential for effectively managing the evolving landscape of *S. aureus* infections and combating antibiotic resistance.

Acknowledgements

The authors would like to acknowledge the financial support from Prime Minister's Research Fellowship (PMRF, ID: 2001303—granted to SA), Scheme for Transformational and Advanced Research in Sciences (STARS), Ministry of Education, Government of India (MoE-STARS/STARS-1/784—granted to SD).

Conflict of interest

The authors declare no conflict of interest.

Appendices and nomenclature

- Antibiotic resistance
- Community-acquired infections
- Culture-based methods
- Cytoplasmic regulators
- Diagnosis
- Endocarditis
- Epidemiology
- Molecular methods
- Pathogenesis
- Pulmonary infections
- Regulatory proteins
- *Staphylococcus aureus*

- Septicemia
- Serological assay
- Two-component systems
- Virulence factors

MRSA	methicillin resistant *S. aureus*
HAIs	Healthcare-Associated Infections
PCR	polymerase chain reaction
TCS	two-component system
Agr	accessory gene regulator
QS	quorum sensing
AIP	autoinducing peptide
PSM	phenol soluble modulin
hld	delta-hemolysin gene
MSSA	methicillin-susceptible *S. aureus*
SSIs	surgical site infections
HIV/AIDS	Human Immunodeficiency Virus/Acquired Immunodeficiency Syndrome
ICUs	intensive care units
HIV	human immunodeficiency virus
COPD	chronic obstructive pulmonary disease
VRSA	vancomycin-resistant *S. aureus*
AMR	antimicrobial resistance
PBP	penicillin-binding protein
SSCmec	Staphylococcal Cassette Chromosome mec
MIC	minimum inhibitory concentration
EIA	enzyme immunoassays
LAMP	loop-mediated isothermal amplification
NAATs	nucleic acid amplification techniques

Author details

Sushama Agarwalla and Suhanya Duraiswamy*
Indian Institute of Technology Hyderabad, Sangareddy, Telangana, India

*Address all correspondence to: suhanya@che.iith.ac.in

References

[1] Arumugam G, Periasamy H, Maneesh Paul S. *Staphylococcus aureus*: Overview of bacteriology, clinical diseases, epidemiology, antibiotic resistance and therapeutic approach. In: Shymaa E, Laura ECA, editors. Frontiers in *Staphylococcus aureus*. London, UK: IntechOpen; 2017. p. Ch. 1w

[2] Gherardi G, Di Bonaventura G, Savini V. Chapter 1—Staphylococcal taxonomy. In: Savini V, editor. Pet-to-Man Travelling Staphylococci. Cambridge, Massachusetts, USA: Academic Press, Elsevier; 2018. pp. 1-10

[3] Glowacka P et al. Virulence factors, pathogenesis and treatment. Polish Journal of Microbiology. 2018;**67**(2):151-161

[4] Kwiecinski JM, Horswill AR. *Staphylococcus aureus* bloodstream infections: Pathogenesis and regulatory mechanisms. Current Opinion in Microbiology. 2020;**53**:51-60

[5] Tong SY et al. *Staphylococcus aureus* infections: Epidemiology, pathophysiology, clinical manifestations, and management. Clinical Microbiology Reviews. 2015;**28**(3):603-661

[6] Samia NI et al. Methicillin-resistant *staphylococcus aureus* nosocomial infection has a distinct epidemiological position and acts as a marker for overall hospital-acquired infection trends. Scientific Reports. 2022;**12**(1):17007

[7] Nakou A, Woodhead M, Torres A. MRSA as a cause of community-acquired pneumonia. The European Respiratory Journal. 2009;**34**(5):1013-1014

[8] Abebe AA, Birhanu AG. Methicillin resistant *Staphylococcus aureus:* Molecular mechanisms underlying drug resistance development and novel strategies to combat. Infection and Drug Resistance. 2023;**16**:7641-7662

[9] Recsei P et al. Regulation of exoprotein gene expression in *Staphylococcus aureus* by agr. Molecular and General Genetics MGG. 1986;**202**:58-61

[10] Davis JS et al. Combination of vancomycin and β-lactam therapy for methicillin-resistant *Staphylococcus aureus* bacteremia: A pilot multicenter randomized controlled trial. Clinical Infectious Diseases. 2016;**62**(2):173-180

[11] Somerville GA, Proctor RA. At the crossroads of bacterial metabolism and virulence factor synthesis in staphylococci. Microbiology and Molecular Biology Reviews Journal. 2009;**73**(2):233-248

[12] Villanueva M et al. Sensory deprivation in *Staphylococcus aureus*. Nature Communications. 2018;**9**(1):523

[13] White MJ et al. Phosphatidylinositol-specific phospholipase C contributes to survival of *Staphylococcus aureus* USA300 in human blood and neutrophils. Infection and Immunity. 2014;**82**(4):1559-1571

[14] Matsuo M et al. Distinct two-component systems in methicillin-resistant *Staphylococcus aureus* can change the susceptibility to antimicrobial agents. The Journal of Antimicrobial Chemotherapy. 2010;**65**(7):1536-1537

[15] Jenul C, Horswill AR. Regulation of *Staphylococcus aureus* virulence. Microbiology Spectrum. 2019;**7**(2):10-1128

[16] Dunman PÁ et al. Transcription profiling-based identification of *Staphylococcus aureus* genes regulated by the agr and/or sarA loci. American Society for Microbiology. 2001: 7341-7353

[17] Cheung GY et al. Role of the accessory gene regulator agr in community-associated methicillin-resistant *Staphylococcus aureus* pathogenesis. Infection and Immunity. 2011;**79**(5):1927-1935

[18] Morfeldt E et al. Activation of alpha-toxin translation in *Staphylococcus aureus* by the trans-encoded antisense RNA, RNAIII. The EMBO Journal. 1995;**14**(18):4569-4577

[19] Wardenburg JB, Patel RJ, Schneewind O. Surface proteins and exotoxins are required for the pathogenesis of *Staphylococcus aureus* pneumonia. Infection and Immunity. 2007;**75**(2):1040-1044

[20] Heyer G et al. *Staphylococcus aureus* agr and sarA functions are required for invasive infection but not inflammatory responses in the lung. Infection and Immunity. 2002;**70**(1):127-133

[21] Geisinger E et al. Inhibition of rot translation by RNAIII, a key feature of agr function. Molecular Microbiology. 2006;**61**(4):1038-1048

[22] Boisset S et al. *Staphylococcus aureus* RNAIII coordinately represses the synthesis of virulence factors and the transcription regulator rot by an antisense mechanism. Genes and Development. 2007;**21**(11):1353-1366

[23] Wright JS III, Jin R, Novick RP. Transient interference with staphylococcal quorum sensing blocks abscess formation. PNAS. 2005;**102**(5):1691-1696

[24] Sharkey Liam KR et al. The two-component system WalKR provides an essential link between cell wall homeostasis and DNA replication in *Staphylococcus aureus*. MBio. 2023;**14**(6):e02262-e02223

[25] Cheung AL et al. Regulation of virulence determinants in vitro and in vivo in *Staphylococcus aureus*. FEMS Immunology and Medical Microbiology. 2004;**40**(1):1-9

[26] Morrison JM et al. The staphylococcal accessory regulator, SarA, is an RNA-binding protein that modulates the mRNA turnover properties of late-exponential and stationary phase *Staphylococcus aureus* cells. Frontiers in Cellular and Infection Microbiology. 2012;**2**:20847

[27] Zielinska AK et al. sarA-mediated repression of protease production plays a key role in the pathogenesis of *S taphylococcus aureus* USA 300 isolates. Molecular Microbiology. 2012;**86**(5):1183-1196

[28] Manna AC, Ray B. Regulation and characterization of rot transcription in *Staphylococcus aureus*. Microbiology. 2007;**153**(5):1538-1545

[29] Kazmierczak MJ, Wiedmann M, Boor KJ. Alternative sigma factors and their roles in bacterial virulence. Microbiology and Molecular Biology Reviews. 2005;**69**(4):527-543

[30] Rodriguez Ayala F, Bartolini M, Grau R. The stress-responsive alternative sigma factor SigB of *Bacillus subtilis* and its relatives: An old friend with new functions. Frontiers in Microbiology. 2020;**11**

[31] Wang B, Muir TW. Regulation of virulence in *Staphylococcus aureus:* Molecular mechanisms and remaining

puzzles. Cell Chemical Biology. 2016;**23**(2):214-224

[32] Novick RP. Autoinduction and signal transduction in the regulation of staphylococcal virulence. Molecular Microbiology. 2003;**48**(6):1429-1449

[33] Martins-Araujo M, Valcárcel J. A guide to one of the genome's best-kept secrets. Molecular Cell. 2008;**31**(6):782-784

[34] Tian M, Day B. Domain switching and host recognition. Molecular Microbiology. 2006;**61**(5):1091-1093

[35] Booth MC et al. Staphylococcal accessory regulator (Sar) in conjunction with agr contributes to *Staphylococcus aureus* virulence in endophthalmitis. Infection and Immunity. 1997;**65**(4):1550-1556

[36] Naber CK. *Staphylococcus aureus* bacteremia: Epidemiology, pathophysiology, and management strategies. Clinical Infectious Diseases. 2009;**48**(Suppl. 4):S231-S237

[37] Coia JE et al. Guidelines for the control and prevention of meticillin-resistant *Staphylococcus aureus* (MRSA) in healthcare facilities. The Journal of Hospital Infection. 2006;**63**:S1-S44

[38] Thimmappa L et al. Risk factors for wound infection caused by methicillin resistant *Staphylococcus aureus* among hospitalized patients: A case control study from a tertiary care hospital in India. African Health Sciences. 2021;**21**(1):286-294

[39] Lee AS et al. Methicillin-resistant *Staphylococcus aureus*. Nature Reviews. Disease Primers. 2018;**4**(1):18033

[40] Cooper T et al. Chapter seven—Invasive devices. In: Percival SL et al., editors. Biofilms in Infection Prevention and Control. Boston: Academic Press; 2014. pp. 91-126

[41] Zukowska A, Zukowski M. Surgical site infection in cardiac surgery. Journal of Clinical Medicine. 2022;**11**(23):6991

[42] González-García S et al. Factors of nasopharynx that favor the colonization and persistence of *Staphylococcus aureus*. In: Zhou X, Zhang Z, editors. Pharynx—Diagnosis and Treatment. London, UK: IntechOpen; 2021. pp. 75-81

[43] Peterson SL. Surgical wound infection. In: Harken AH, Moore EE, editors. Abernathy's Surgical Secrets. 6th ed. Philadelphia: Mosby; 2009. pp. 68-72

[44] Bucataru A et al. Factors contributing to surgical site infections: A comprehensive systematic review of etiology and risk factors. Clinics and Practice. 2023;**14**(1):52-68

[45] Tam K, Torres VJ. *Staphylococcus aureus* secreted toxins and extracellular enzymes. Microbiology Spectrum. 2019;**7**(2):10-1128

[46] Thorlacius-Ussing L et al. Age-dependent increase in incidence of *Staphylococcus aureus* bacteremia, Denmark, 2008-2015. Emerging Infectious Diseases. 2019;**25**(5):875-882

[47] Ciabattini A et al. Vaccination in the elderly: The challenge of immune changes with aging. Seminars in Immunology. 2018;**40**:83-94

[48] Marimuthu Ragavan R, Narasingam A. Drug-resistant bacterial infections in HIV patients. In: Samuel O, editor. Advances in HIV and AIDS Control. London, UK: IntechOpen; 2018. p. Ch. 5

[49] Darwitz BP, Genito CJ, Thurlow LR. Triple threat: How diabetes results in

worsened bacterial infections. Infection and Immunity. 2024:e00509-e00523

[50] Calvo M, Stefani S, Migliorisi G. Bacterial infections in intensive care units: Epidemiological and microbiological aspects. Antibiotics. 2024;**13**(3):238

[51] Parameswaran GI, Murphy TF. Infections in chronic lung diseases. Infectious Disease Clinics of North America. 2007;**21**(3):673-695, viii

[52] Espi M et al. Chronic kidney disease-associated immune dysfunctions: Impact of protein-bound uremic retention solutes on immune cells. Toxins. 2020;**12**(5):300

[53] Ceccarelli F et al. *Staphylococcus aureus* nasal carriage and autoimmune diseases: From pathogenic mechanisms to disease susceptibility and phenotype. International Journal of Molecular Sciences. 2019;**20**(22):5624

[54] Roberts MB, Fishman JA. Immunosuppressive agents and infectious risk in transplantation: Managing the "net state of immunosuppression". Clinical Infectious Diseases. 2021;**73**(7):e1302-e1317

[55] Alsolami A et al. Community-acquired methicillin-resistant *Staphylococcus aureus* in hospitals: Age-specificity and potential zoonotic–zooanthroponotic transmission dynamics. Diagnostics. 2023;**13**(12):2089

[56] Marks LR et al. *Staphylococcus aureus* injection drug use-associated bloodstream infections are propagated by community outbreaks of diverse lineages. Communication and Medicine. 2021;**1**(1):52

[57] Mathur P. Hand hygiene: Back to the basics of infection control. The Indian Journal of Medical Research. 2011;**134**(5):611-620

[58] Linz MS et al. Clinical impact of *Staphylococcus aureus* skin and soft tissue infections. Antibiotics (Basel). 2023;**12**(3):557

[59] Mariani F, Galvan EM. *Staphylococcus aureus* in polymicrobial skinand soft tissue infections: Impact of inter-species interactionsin disease outcome. Antibiotics. 2023;**12**(7):1164

[60] McCaig LF et al. *Staphylococcus aureus*-associated skin and soft tissue infections in ambulatory care. Emerging Infectious Diseases. 2006;**12**(11):1715-1723

[61] Alvarez-Uria G et al. Intra-abscess administration of antibiotics through ultrasound-guided percutaneous catheter for the treatment of pyogenic liver abscess. Journal of Clinical and Diagnostic Research. 2013;**7**(8):1698-1699

[62] Clebak KT, Malone MA. Skin infections. Primary Care: Clinics in Office Practice. 2018;**45**(3):433-454

[63] Sullivan T, de Barra E. Diagnosis and management of cellulitis. Clinical Medicine (London, England). 2018;**18**(2):160-163

[64] Urish KL, Cassat JE. *Staphylococcus aureus* osteomyelitis: Bone, bugs, and surgery. Infection and Immunity. 2020;**88**(7):10-1128

[65] Long B, Koyfman A, Gottlieb M. Evaluation and management of septic arthritis and its mimics in the emergency department. The Western Journal of Emergency Medicine. 2019;**20**(2):331-341

[66] Mathews CJ et al. Management of septic arthritis: A systematic review.

Annals of the Rheumatic Diseases. 2007;**66**(4):440-445

[67] Brooks WA. 42—Bacterial pneumonia. In: Ryan ET et al., editors. Hunter's Tropical Medicine and Emerging Infectious Diseases. 10th ed. London: Elsevier; 2020. pp. 446-453

[68] Ragle BE, Karginov VA, Bubeck Wardenburg J. Prevention and treatment of *Staphylococcus aureus* pneumonia with a beta-cyclodextrin derivative. Antimicrobial Agents and Chemotherapy. 2010;**54**(1):298-304

[69] Chinemerem Nwobodo D et al. Antibiotic resistance: The challenges and some emerging strategies for tackling a global menace. Journal of Clinical Laboratory Analysis. 2022;**36**(9):e24655

[70] Shaw SP. Chapter 176—β-lactam antimicrobials. In: Silverstein DC, Hopper K, editors. Small Animal Critical Care Medicine. 2nd ed. St. Louis: W.B. Saunders; 2015. pp. 928-929

[71] Barreiro C et al. Chapter 5—Beta-lactam antibiotics. In: Dhara AK, Nayak AK, Chattopadhyay D, editors. Antibiotics—Therapeutic Spectrum and Limitations. Cambridge, Massachusetts, USA: Academic Press, Elsevier; 2023. pp. 89-122

[72] Kang C-I et al. Clinical practice guidelines for the antibiotic treatment of community-acquired urinary tract infections. Journal of Infection and Chemotherapy. 2018;**50**(1):67-100

[73] Leekha S, Terrell CL, Edson RS. General principles of antimicrobial therapy. Mayo Clinic Proceedings. 2011;**86**(2):156-167

[74] Davies J, Davies D. Origins and evolution of antibiotic resistance. Microbiology and Molecular Biology Reviews. 2010;**74**(3):417-433

[75] Malachowa N, DeLeo FR. Mobile genetic elements of *staphylococcus aureus*. Cellular and Molecular Life Sciences. 2010;**67**(18):3057-3071

[76] Saber T et al. Methicillin- and vancomycin-resistant *Staphylococcus aureus* from humans and ready-to-eat meat: Characterization of antimicrobial resistance and biofilm formation ability. Frontiers in Microbiology. 2022;**12**:735494

[77] Wright GD. Mechanisms of resistance to antibiotics. Current Opinion in Chemical Biology. 2003;**7**(5):563-569

[78] Deurenberg RH, Stobberingh EE. The evolution of *Staphylococcus aureus*. Infection, Genetics and Evolution. 2008;**8**(6):747-763

[79] Cong Y, Yang S, Rao X. Vancomycin resistant *Staphylococcus aureus* infections: A review of case updating and clinical features. Journal of Advanced Research. 2020;**21**:169-176

[80] Chandler L. Chapter 20—Challenges in clinical microbiology testing. In: Dasgupta A, Sepulveda JL, editors. Accurate Results in the Clinical Laboratory. San Diego: Elsevier; 2013. pp. 315-326

[81] Opota O et al. Blood culture-based diagnosis of bacteraemia: State of the art. Clinical Microbiology and Infection. 2015;**21**(4):313-322

[82] Doškař J et al. Molecular diagnostics of *Staphylococcus aureus*. In: Detection of Bacteria, Viruses, Parasites and Fungi. Dordrecht: Springer Netherlands; 2010

[83] Wu S et al. A review of the methods for detection of *Staphylococcus aureus* enterotoxins. Toxins. 2016;**8**(7):176

[84] Steinbach WJ, Shetty AK. Use of the diagnostic bacteriology laboratory:

A practical review for the clinician. Postgraduate Medical Journal. 2001;**77**(905):148-156

[85] Shanson DC. Chapter 1—Classification and pathogenicity of microbes. In: Shanson DC, editor. Microbiology in Clinical Practice. 2nd ed. Oxford, UK: Butterworth-Heinemann, Elsevier; 1989. pp. 3-32

[86] Grüner BM et al. Characterization of a catalase-negative methicillin-resistant *Staphylococcus aureus* strain. Journal of Clinical Microbiology. 2007;**45**(8):2684-2685

[87] Alipour F, Ahmadi M, Javadi S. Evaluation of different methods to detect methicillin resistance in *Staphylococcus aureus* (MRSA). Journal of Infection and Public Health. 2014;7(3):186-191

[88] He J. Chapter 5.1—Practical guide to ELISA development. In: Wild D, editor. The Immunoassay Handbook. 4th ed. Oxford: Elsevier; 2013. pp. 381-393

[89] Crosby HA, Kwiecinski J, Horswill AR. *Staphylococcus aureus* aggregation and coagulation mechanisms, and their function in host-pathogen interactions. Advances in Applied Microbiology. 2016;**96**:1-41

[90] Yang S, Rothman RE. PCR-based diagnostics for infectious diseases: Uses, limitations, and future applications in acute-care settings. The Lancet Infectious Diseases. 2004;**4**(6):337-348

[91] Liu Y, Zhang J, Ji Y. PCR-based approaches for the detection of clinical methicillin-resistant *Staphylococcus aureus*. The Open Microbiology Journal. 2016;**10**:45-56

[92] Costa A-M, Kay I, Palladino S. Rapid detection of mecA and nuc genes in staphylococci by real-time multiplex polymerase chain reaction. Diagnostic Microbiology and Infectious Disease. 2005;**51**(1):13-17

[93] Carroll KC. Rapid diagnostics for methicillin-resistant *Staphylococcus aureus*. Molecular Diagnosis and Therapy. 2008;**12**(1):15-24

[94] Palavecino EL. Rapid methods for detection of MRSA in clinical specimens. In: Ji Y, editor. Methicillin-Resistant *Staphylococcus Aureus* (MRSA) Protocols. Totowa, NJ: Humana Press; 2014. pp. 71-83

[95] Li Y et al. Loop-mediated isothermal amplification (LAMP): A novel rapid detection platform for pathogens. Microbial Pathogenesis. 2017;**107**:54-61

[96] Khosravi AD et al. The application of the loop-mediated isothermal amplification method for rapid detection of methicillin-resistant *Staphylococcus aureus*. New Microbes New Infections. 2022;**45**:100960

[97] Goyal PA et al. Revolutionizing medical microbiology: How molecular and genomic approaches are changing diagnostic techniques. Cureus. 2023;**15**(10):e47106

[98] Alhammad L et al. The impact of laboratory automation on efficiency and accuracy in healthcare settings. International Journal of Community Medicine and Public Health. 2023;**11**:1347